DIAGNOSTIC PICTURE TESTS IN

GENERAL MEDICINE

Michael Zatouroff
FRCP Lond., DCH

Physician, Harley Street, London.
Honorary Senior Lecturer in Medicine,
Academic Department of Medicine,
Royal Free Hospital, London.

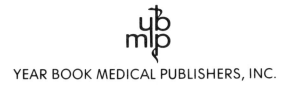

YEAR BOOK MEDICAL PUBLISHERS, INC.

Titles in this series, published or being developed, include:

Diagnostic Picture Tests in Pediatrics
Picture Tests in Human Anatomy
Diagnostic Picture Tests in Oral Medicine
Diagnostic Picture Tests in Orthopedics
Diagnostic Picture Tests in Infectious Diseases
Diagnostic Picture Tests in Dermatology
Diagnostic Picture Tests in Ophthalmology
Diagnostic Picture Tests in Rheumatology
Diagnostic Picture Tests in Obstetrics/Gynecology
Diagnostic Picture Tests in Clinical Neurology
Diagnostic Picture Tests in Injury in Sport
Diagnostic Picture Tests in General Surgery
Diagnostic Picture Tests in General Medicine
Diagnostic Picture Tests in Pediatric Dentistry
Diagnostic Picture Tests in Dentistry
Picture Tests in Embryology

Copyright © M. Zatouroff, 1988
First published 1988 by Wolfe Medical Publications Ltd
Printed by W.S. Cowell Ltd, Ipswich, England

Library of Congress Cataloging-in-Publication Data

Zatouroff, M.
    Diagnostic picture tests in general medicine
    Includes index.
    ISBN 0 8151 9884 1

    1. Diagnosis—Examinations, questions, etc. 2. Diagnosis—
Atlases. I. Title.
    [DNLM: 1. Diagnosis—atlases. 2. Diagnosis—examination
questions. 3. Medicine—atlases. 4. Medicine—examination
questions. WB 18 Z38d].
RC71.Z35   1988
616.075—dc19
DNLM/DLC   87–29437
for Library of Congress   CIP

Preface

This collection of clinical photographs represents an eclectic selection covering a broad spectrum of general internal medicine. The usual photographs of physical signs can be dull and repetitive. Problem pictures are more fun. Thus, my own approach to teaching with slides has been one of emphasising data collection from the photograph, hypothesising and confirming the hypothesis by further analysis and then using the frequency of occurrence as a balance. This allows one to produce common answers first and abstruse answers second.

Each picture/X-ray should make a point and a question is asked at an elementary and a more advanced level, some of which may be difficult to answer unless the abnormality in the photograph has first been recognised. A picture may be of a physical sign but the question may refer to a relation or be unconnected to the actual photograph, the connection requiring some lateral thinking. The questions are meant to increase one's ability to observe, to stimulate and teach. Seeing and thinking is the message, but with considerable emphasis on enjoyment. The pictures can be approached at random but the text of the answers should be read a second time with the photograph for direct reference.

No apology for this lateral approach is necessary for it will encourage a wide-ranging search of the memory for associations in medicine. This can be important when faced with unusual presentations of disease.

All of the photographs, with the exception of numbers 160, 172-174, 201-203 and 209 were taken by the author, either with a Leica R3/R4 and a 60mm Macro Elmar lens by available light or with a Nikon F3 and a Medi-Nikkor lens on Kodachrome 25 reversal film.

Acknowledgements

My thanks to Sir Richard Bayliss, FRCP for providing illustrations 201, 202, 203, 209 and to Dr Imrich Sarkany, FRCP for 160, 172, 173, 174.

The assistance of my secretary Shelley Lever was greatly appreciated.

For Diana

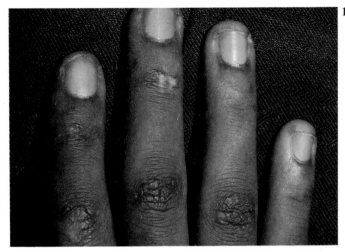

1 A 23-year-old girl complained of extreme muscle tenderness and weakness.
(a) What physical signs might be seen in the skin?
(b) What other investigations are indicated?
(c) What is the diagnosis? Give two associated groups of disease.

2 (a) In which genetically determined disease is this abnormality (right finger) seen?
(b) In which disease does this sign appear after treatment?
(c) Give two diseases with characteristic bony changes.

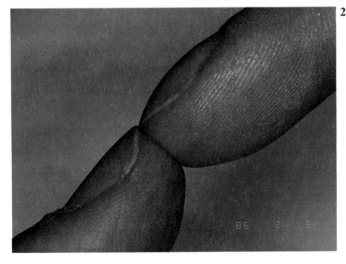

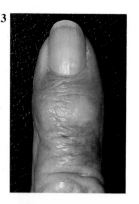

3 (a) What is the cause of this physical sign?
(b) Give three characteristic sites that are affected in the hand.

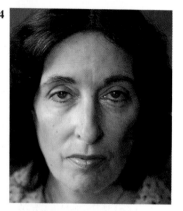

4 A 45-year-old woman underwent cataract extraction six years ago.
(a) What is the diagnosis?
(b) Give four causes of the bilateral physical signs shown.
(c) In this patient, what are the risks of general anaesthesia?
(d) Why may she dislike cold weather?

5 A 23-year-old woman had fever, arthralgia and a skin rash occurring at menstruation.
(a) What is the diagnosis?
(b) What is the differential diagnosis?

6 A man complained of breast enlargement.

(a) What drug may have been prescribed in the past four months and why?

(b) What physical signs are apparent?

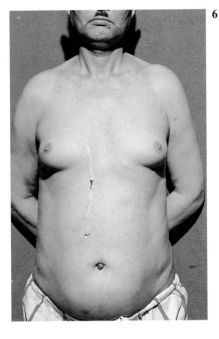

7 A 60-year-old woman presented with occipital headache, early morning lethargy and a rash.

(a) What blood test is indicated?

(b) What is the differential diagnosis?

(c) What condition has now developed?

(d) Give three conditions that may be preceded by this rash.

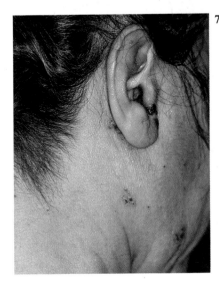

8 A Pakistani child in northern England presented with weakness and pain in the legs.
(a) What are the physical signs?
(b) What are the possible causes?
(c) What are the underlying reasons?
(d) What is the diagnosis?

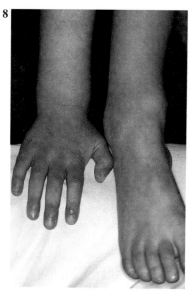

9 A young boy presented with bellyache and a painful hip.
(a) What is the diagnosis?
(b) What advice would you offer the anaesthetist if an operation is necessary?
(c) What is the likely organism involved?

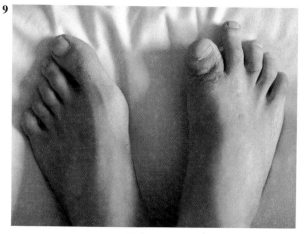

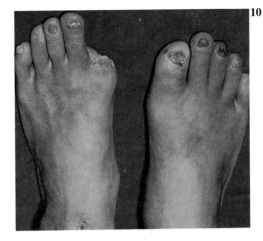

10 This 23-year-old Chinese cook is a heavy smoker and suffers from Raynaud's phenomenon in the hands and pain on walking.
(a) What are the physical signs?
(b) What is the diagnosis?

11 A hypertensive 50-year-old man was admitted as an emergency. You see him two weeks later.
(a) What are the physical signs?
(b) What is the diagnosis?

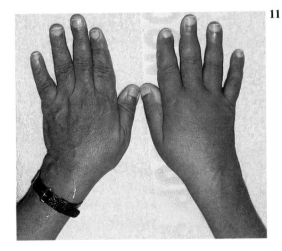

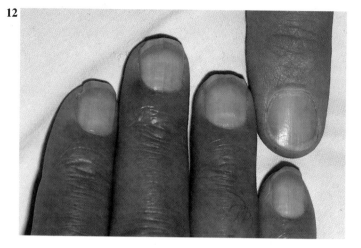

12 (a) What urine test is indicated when this nail appearance is seen?
(b) What diagnoses does the nail colour suggest?

13 A young fashion model returned from a photographic trip to Nigeria with a high fever.
(a) What physical sign is shown?
(b) With what may it be associated?
(c) What is the diagnosis?
(d) What is the differential diagnosis?

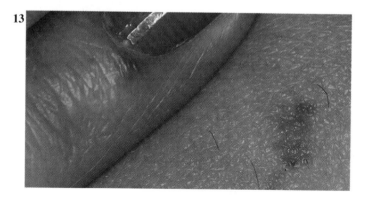

14 Two iatrogenic physical signs are shown; one is an anachronism, and one is inflammatory.
(a) What are they?
(b) What is the diagnosis?

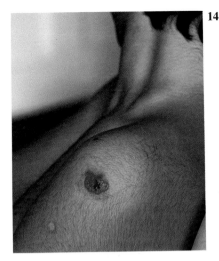

15, 16 The patient is gazing at the ceiling (**15**). He is then asked to look at an object placed level with the bridge of the nose (**16**). Note that the pupils have constricted.
(a) Give three causes for failure to observe this reaction.
(b) What infectious disease may produce paralysis of accommodation?

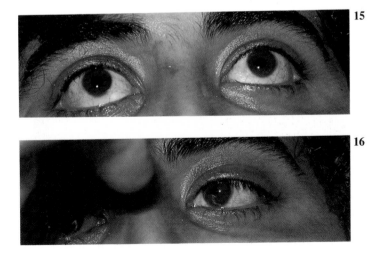

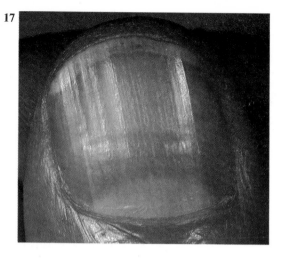

17 (a) What minor nail changes are noted in this thumb nail?
(b) What is their significance?

18–21 This elderly man complained of double vision and pain over the eyes.
(a) What physical signs are noted?
(b) Give four possible causes.
(c) Which is the least likely and why?
(d) What is the diagnosis?

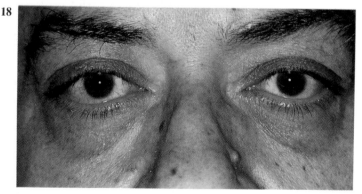

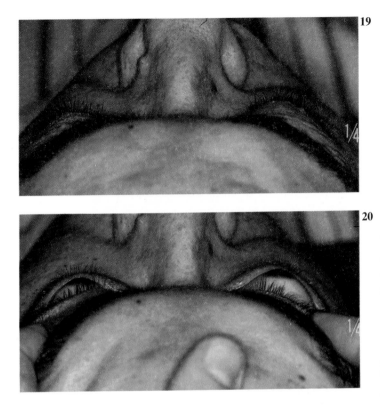

19

20

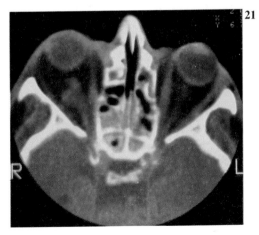

21

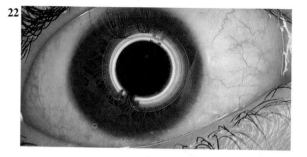

22 There is a brown ring at the junction with the cornea in a pharmacist admitted to hospital having vomited blood.
(a) What abnormality is seen in the eye?
(b) What physical sign may be found in the abdomen and the arms?

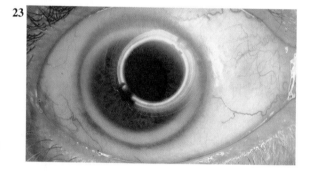

23 (a) What is the diagnosis and its relevance at 60 years and 30 years?
(b) What other clinical signs would you look for?

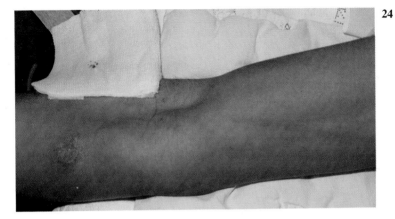

24 This 11-year-old boy presents with anorexia. His grandmother was admitted to hospital with weight loss of three months' duration.
(a) What may be found in the axilla?
(b) What was wrong with the grandmother?
(c) What is the significance of the physical signs?

25 A young male complained of diplopia of recent onset.
(a) What are the physical signs?
(b) What clinical test will confirm your suspicions?
(c) Why is the right eye injected?
(d) What are the common causes of this condition?
(e) What is the diagnosis?

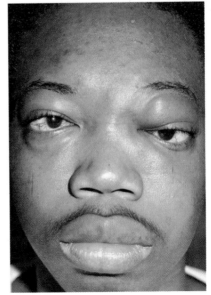

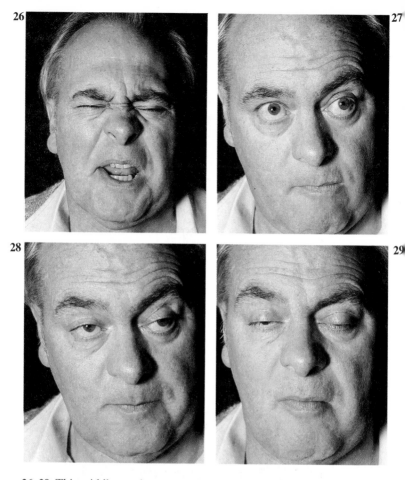

26–29 This middle-aged man complained of increasing difficulty in chewing during the course of a meal and had bilateral complete ptosis after three minutes of sustained upward gaze (**27–29**). In **26** he is responding to the command 'screw up your eyes and show your teeth'.

(a) Give four causes of bilateral ptosis.

(b) Give reasons for your final diagnosis.

30 This woman suffered from recurrent severe headaches, and presented with these physical signs.
(a) What is the cause of the signs?
(b) What is the differential diagnosis?

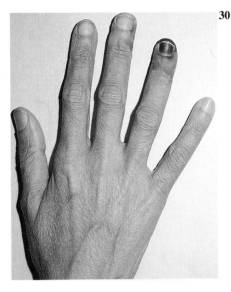

30

31 A 52-year-old woman with a nine-year history of Raynaud's phenomenon presented with difficulty in swallowing solid food.
(a) What is wrong with the hands and fingers?
(b) Give four other systems that may be affected in this condition.

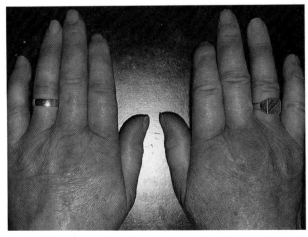

31

32

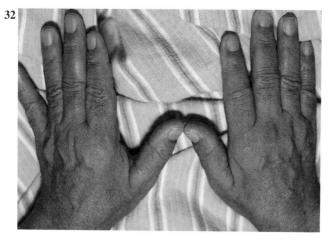

32 (a) What physical sign is seen in both hands?
(b) What would you look for in the face?

33

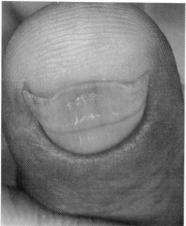

33 (a) What common disorder leads to nails of this configuration?
(b) What are the symptoms traditionally associated with it?
(c) What is the diagnosis?

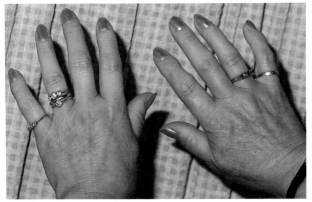

34 A 60-year-old housewife complained of pain in the knees after exercise.
(a) What is the diagnosis?
(b) What two cardinal signs are shown?
(c) What other feature may be present?

35 (a) What might you find on examining the hand and arm?
(b) What is the diagnosis?

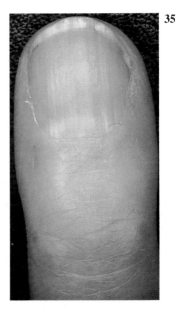

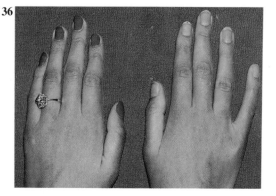

36 A young girl presented with a vascular accident secondary to the contraceptive pill.
(a) Which is the abnormal hand and why?
(b) What may be seen in the affected limb?
(c) What were the X-ray signs?

37 A heavy smoker complained of breathlessness.
(a) What is the abnormal appearance?
(b) What is the cause?

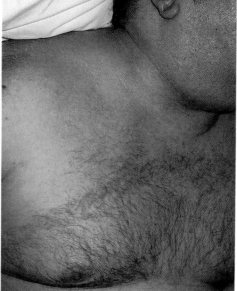

38 (a) What is the condition?
(b) Give four causes of a similar appearance.

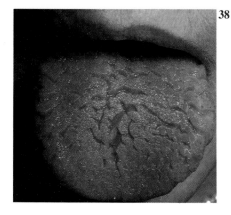

39 A 60-year-old man presented with occipital headache, shoulder stiffness and low grade fever.
(a) What physical sign is seen?
(b) What investigation is relevant?
(c) What may be found on biopsy?
(d) What diagnosis may be made?

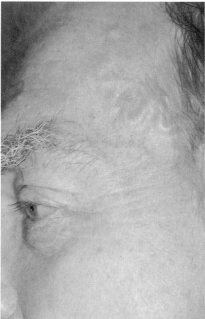

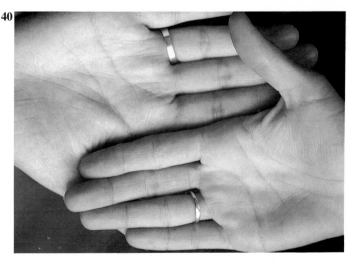

40 A man presents with lethargy, cold intolerance and weight gain; his hand and a control are shown.
(a) What is the physical sign and the diagnosis?
(b) What is the mechanism?
(c) Give three causes of the sign.

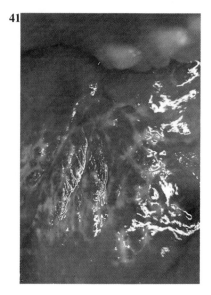

41 The buccal mucosa of a man with pruritus is shown.
(a) What is the diagnosis?
(b) What other conditions may lead to confusion?
(c) What other parts of the body would you examine?
(d) How else might this appearance be produced?

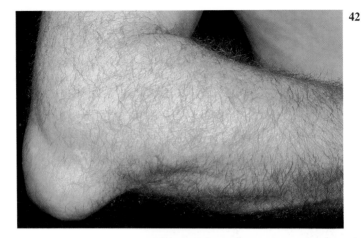

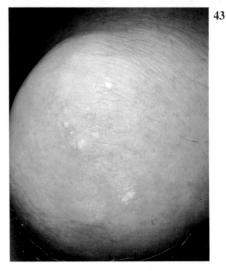

42, 43 (a) What is the physical sign?
(b) Why is it not what it appears?
(c) What is the diagnosis?
(d) Where else would you examine?

44

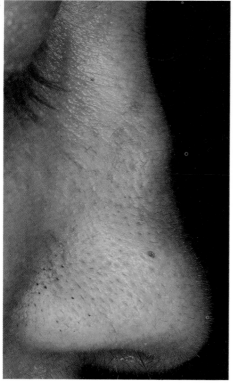

44 Depression of the nasal bridge began at 35 years of age, associated with fever and soreness of the larynx; there is inflammation and softening of the cartilage.

(a) What is the diagnosis?

(b) What other sites may be affected?

(c) Give two other causes for this physical sign.

45 (a) Give two physical signs.

(b) Give six causes of the second physical sign.

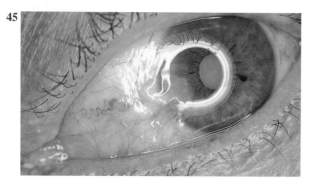

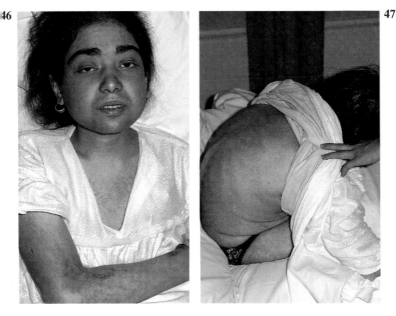

46–48 This patient has pain in the back, weight loss and polydipsia.
(a) What is the diagnosis? (There are three signs in **46**, two signs in **47**, and two signs in **48**.)
(b) What may happen after treatment?

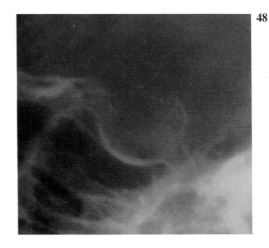

49

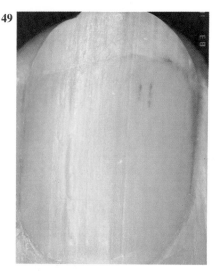

49 (a) What is the significance of the physical sign?
(b) Give three causes.
(c) What is the likely diagnosis from the physical signs seen?

50

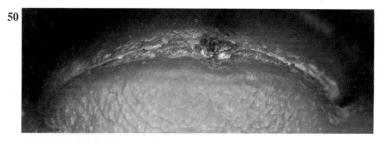

51

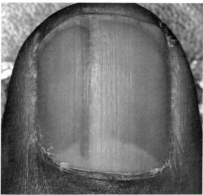

50, 51 A young man presented with hypotension and increasing lethargy.
(a) What is the change in the nail?
(b) Could it relate to his complaint?
(c) What other possibilities are there?

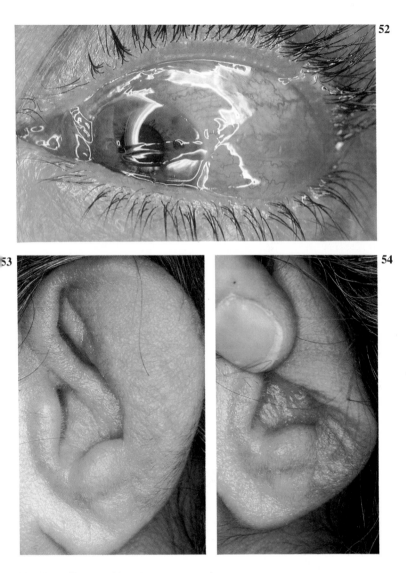

52–54 A 45-year-old woman presented with a three-week history of red eyes and painful anterior chest wall and ears.
(a) What is the diagnosis?
(b) What has happened to the eye and ear?
(c) What other physical signs may be present?

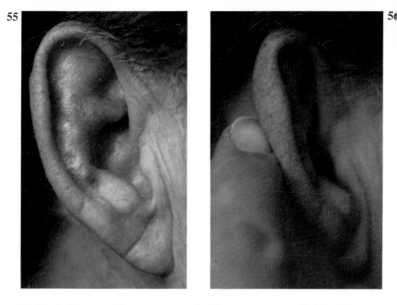

55, 56 A 45-year-old man presented with severe osteoarthritis of the hips and knees.
(a) What is the underlying condition?
(b) What change may be seen in his urine if stood overnight?

57 A male West African's nails with a pigment change. Give five causes of pigment change.

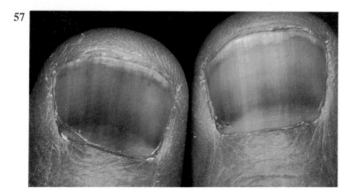

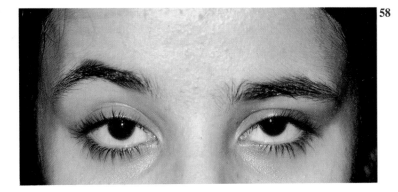

58 A young girl complained of drooping of the left eyelid.
(a) What is the diagnosis?
(b) How do you analyse ptosis?

59 A 40-year-old woman complained of pain in the hands at night.
(a) What is shown?
(b) What muscle is affected?
(c) What is its nerve and segmental supply?
(d) What is the diagnosis?
(e) Give four associated endocrine conditions.

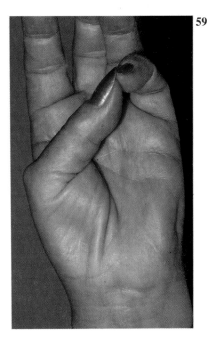

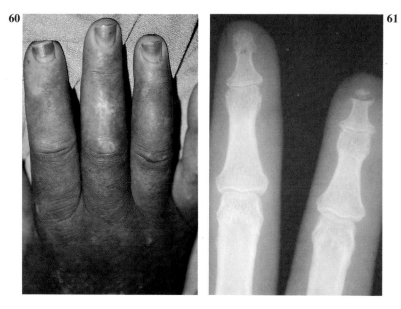

60, 61 A woman presented with breathlessness.
(a) Give three typical visible signs.
(b) Give three variants of this condition.
(c) Give five systems affected by this condition.

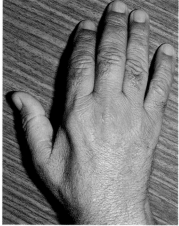

62 A 50-year-old cigarette smoker presented with a numb medial side of the hand.
(a) What physical sign is shown?
(b) What pupillary abnormality was present?
(c) Which nerves and segments are affected?
(d) What is the diagnosis?

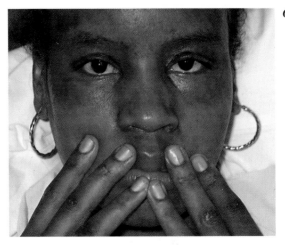

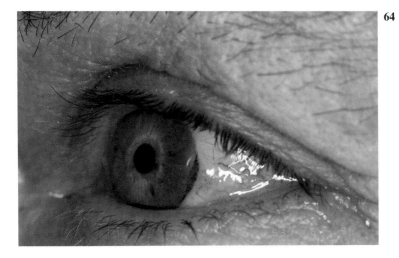

63 A young woman presented with a recent onset of difficulty on trying to climb stairs.
(a) What is the diagnosis?
(b) Give four diseases that may present in this manner.
(c) Give four typical features as seen here.
(d) What associated condition should be excluded?

64 (a) What is the sign?
(b) Give three differential diagnoses.

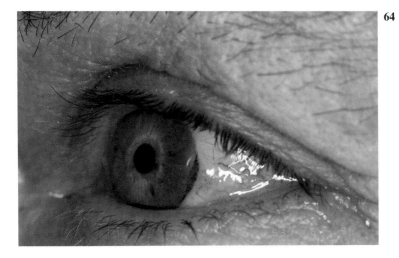

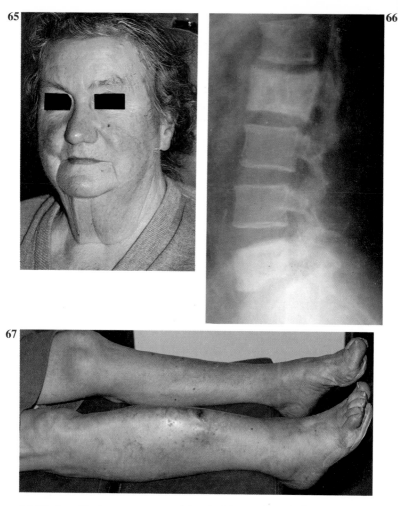

65–67 An elderly woman complained of increasing deafness, breathlessness and an aching lower leg.

(a) What did examination of the heart disclose?
(b) What may cause skull enlargement?
(c) What are the commonest manifestations of this condition?
(d) How do the legs differ on palpation?
(e) What complications may occur locally; generally?
(f) What does the X-ray of the spine show?

68 A male presents with a cough.
(a) What physical sign is seen?
(b) What components of the syndrome are *not* seen?
(c) What clues are present to the level of the lesion?
(d) What is the diagnosis?

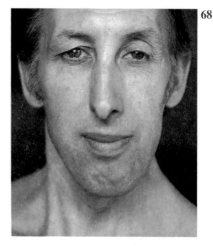

68

69 A 69-year-old male with a history of bilateral renal colic presented with vomiting and lethargy.
(a) What is wrong with his hand?
(b) What else did he have?

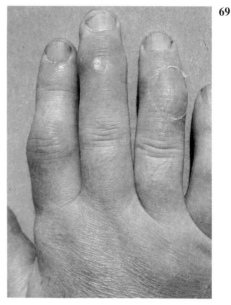

69

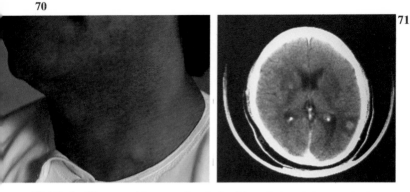

70–73 At 35 years old, a previously healthy, Gujerati (vegetarian) male had his first grand mal epileptic fit.
(a) What is the significance of the clinical photograph?
(b) What are the inconsistencies?
(c) What may be found on general examination, CT scan, X-ray and biopsy?

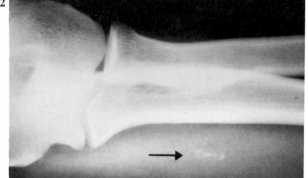

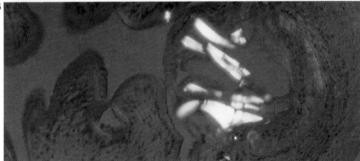

74 (a) What does the X-ray show?
(b) Give seven causes of calcification in cartilage.
(c) What is the diagnosis?

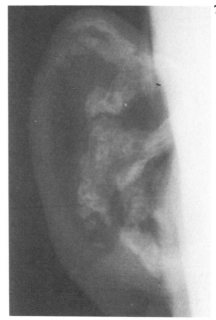

75 (a) What is the physical sign?
(b) Give two other associated sites.

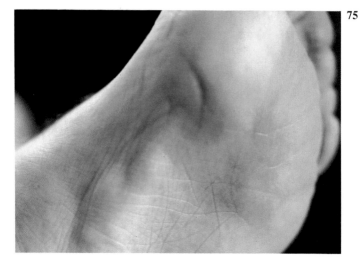

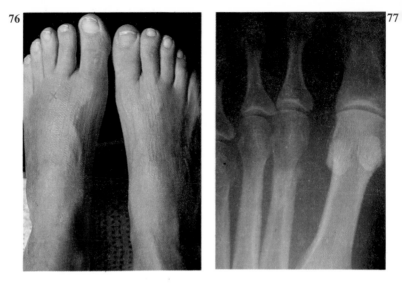

76, 77 After a walking tour this patient complained of pain in the left forefoot. Give four causes in order of probability.

78 (a) What is the physical sign?
(b) Give four associations for it.

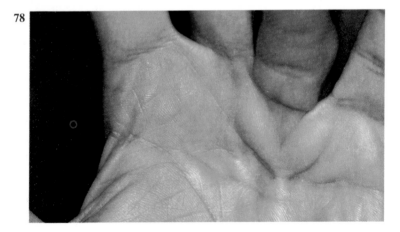

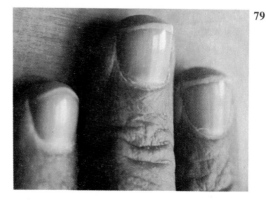

79 (a) What is the change seen in this 45-year-old man?
(b) Give two causes.
(c) What might be found in the urine?

80 This man's grand-daughter presented with raised tender lumps on her shins.
(a) What is the diagnosis in the girl?
(b) What is the diagnosis in the man and what structures are affected?

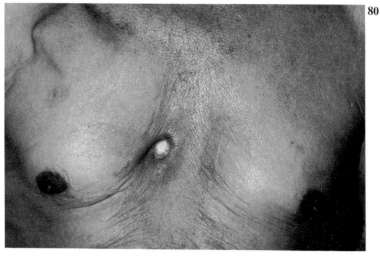

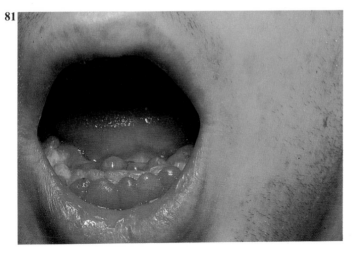

81 (a) What is the diagnosis?
(b) Give two differential diagnoses.
(c) Give three causes of this appearance.

82 A mildly hypertensive football fan presented early on Sunday morning.
(a) What is the likely diagnosis?
(b) Give three precipitating causes.

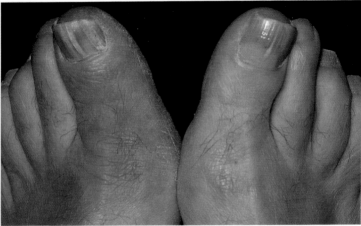

83 A young woman complained of sweating and pains in the hands.
(a) Why does she sweat excessively?
(b) Why does she have hand pain?
(c) Give five conditions presenting with excess sweating.

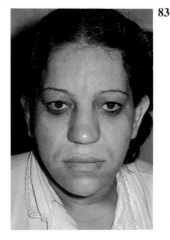

83

84 A woman was brought unconscious to casualty; careful general observation discloses this lesion.
(a) What immediate action would you take?
(b) What is the diagnosis?
(c) Give two differential diagnoses.

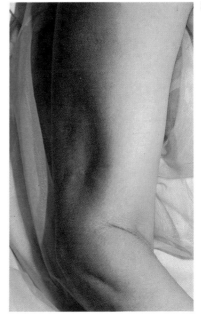

84

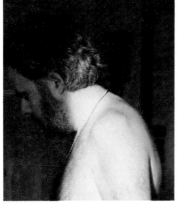 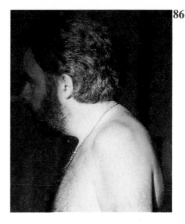

85, 86 A middle-aged male, displaying his range of flexion and extension of the neck, complained of intermittent loose stools, red eyes and backache.
(a) What is the diagnosis?
(b) Give five features of the condition.
(c) Why may he complain of chest pain?
(d) Why is driving a hazard?

87 (a) Observe five physical signs.
(b) Give two differential diagnoses.
(c) Give three nail changes in this condition.
(d) What is the diagnosis?

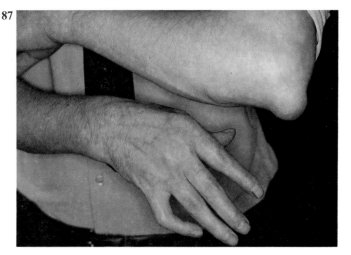

88 This patient complained of polyuria.
(a) Give six features of this condition.
(b) Give four causes.
(c) What is the diagnosis?

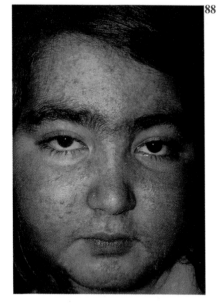

89 This young girl presented with migraine.
(a) Give two physical signs.
(b) Give three causes for each sign.
(c) What is the diagnosis?

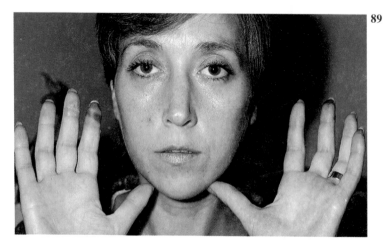

90

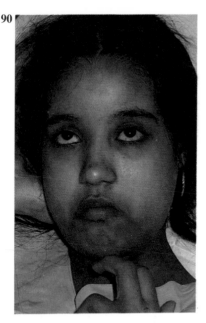

90 An 18-year-old girl presented with nausea, vomiting and renal failure with a spasm of the external ocular muscles.
(a) What is the diagnosis?
(b) What has occurred?
(c) Give three causes of this appearance.

91 (a) Why is it difficult to elicit the knee tendon reflex?
(b) What is unusual in the figure?
(c) Give four associated features.
(d) What is the diagnosis?

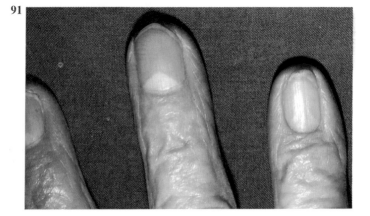

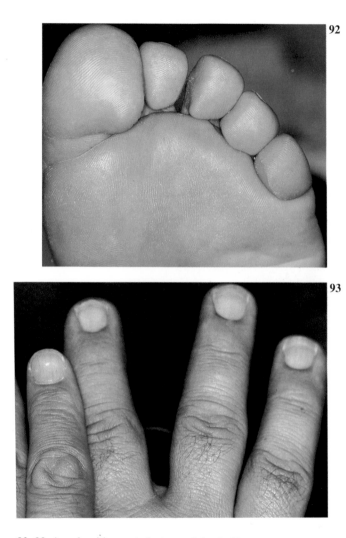

92, 93 A male with sweaty feet complained of impotence.
(a) What is the diagnosis?
(b) What physical signs are seen in the extremities?

94

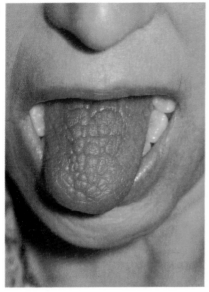

94 This woman has difficulty in public speaking.
(a) What appearance may be seen in: the eye; the joints; the lymph glands; the abdomen; the blood film?
(b) What is the diagnosis?

95 A middle-aged woman presented with dysphagia and stiff fingers.
(a) What is the diagnosis?
(b) Give six presentations of this condition.

95

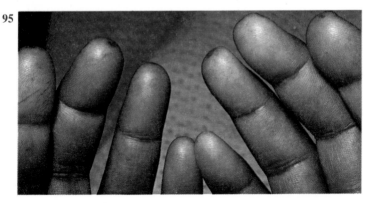

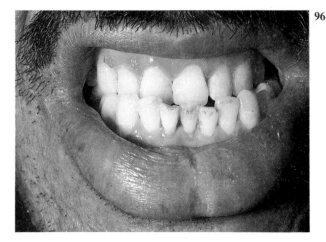

96 This male complained of fatigue.
(a) Give two physical changes seen.
(b) Give three rheumatological manifestations of this condition.
(c) What is the diagnosis?

97 A 30-year-old man whose father died suddenly aged 40 years.
(a) What other physical signs would you look for?
(b) What is the most likely diagnosis?

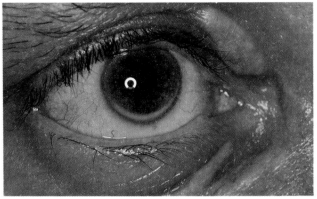

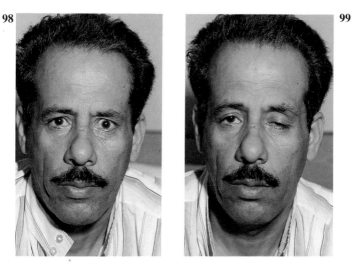

98, 99 A male complained of 'difficulty in chewing coming on during a meal'.
(a) What has happened between **98** and **99**?
(b) Give two associated diseases.
(c) Give two associated drugs.
(d) What is the diagnosis?

100 This woman complained of looseness of the stools, right-sided drooping of the eyelid, and weight loss.
(a) Give two interpretations of this clinical picture.
(b) What is the diagnosis?

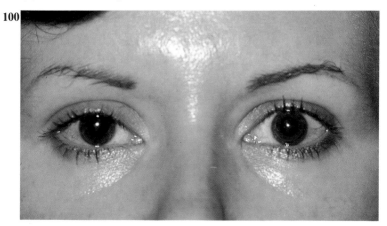

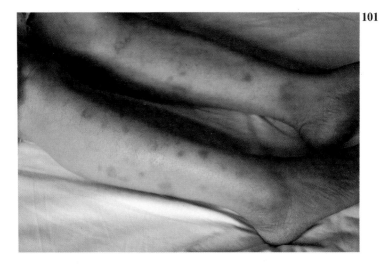

101, 102 A woman complained of fever and pain in the knees (the ulnar border of the arms and shins are shown).

(a) What is the diagnosis?

(b) Give five common and five less common causes.

(c) Give the most important investigations.

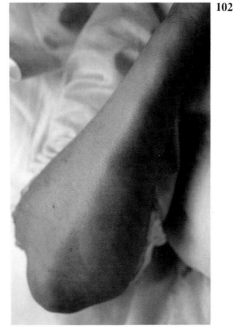

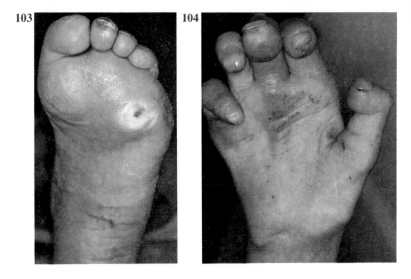

103, 104 The limbs of an uncomplaining Turkish waiter are shown.
(a) Give three causes of the foot appearance.
(b) What nerves are affected in the hand?
(c) What is the diagnosis?

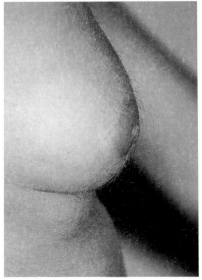

105 (a) Give seven conditions causing this man's appearance.
(b) What drugs other than oestrogens cause this appearance?
(c) What is the diagnosis?

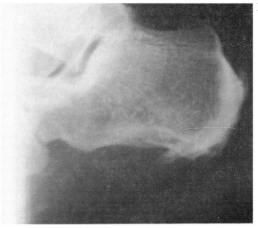

106 A middle-aged woman presented with painful heels.
(a) What can you note on the X-ray?
(b) Give four diseases associated with this appearance.

107 (a) What abnormality may be seen: on examining the right eye; on the chest X-ray?
(b) What is the diagnosis?

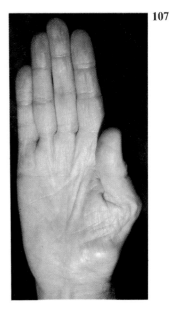

108 (a) What abnormality is seen?
(b) Give five causes.

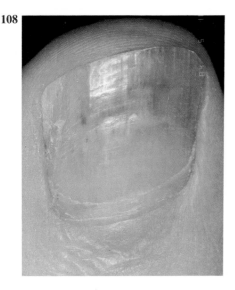

109 (a) What facts can be deduced from observing this man's abdomen?
(b) What is the most likely diagnosis?

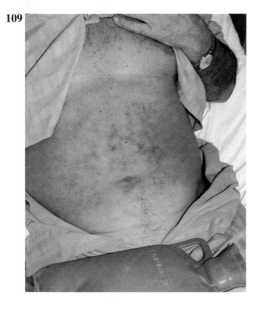

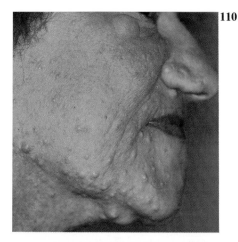

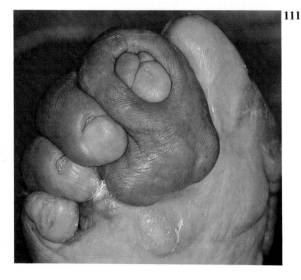

110, 111 This patient complained of enlargement of the feet.
(a) What causes the facial appearance?
(b) Why are the feet enlarging?
(c) Give other manifestations of the condition.
(d) What is the diagnosis?

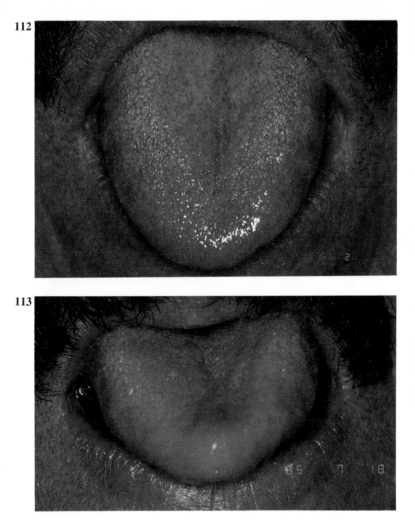

112,113 A 30-year-old male presents with a hoarse voice; the picture at presentation (**112**) and 3 months later (**113**) is shown. What is the diagnosis?

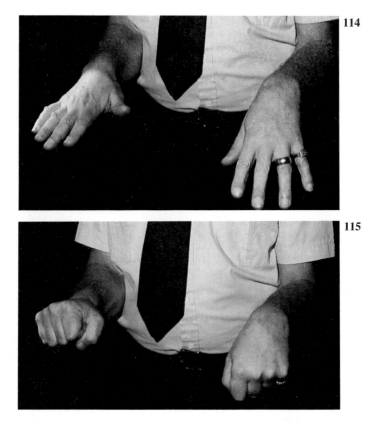

114, 115 This diabetic awoke unable to extend the left wrist or the fingers.
(a) What nerve is affected?
(b) Give four sites of damage and state how they may be differentiated.

116

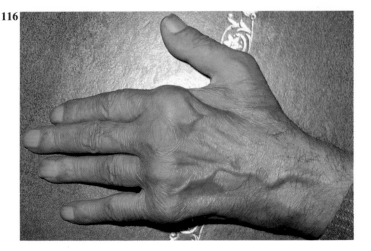

116 (a) What is the diagnosis?
(b) Outline an approach to wasting of small muscles of the hand.
(c) Which muscles are wasted?

117 A 60-year-old opium addict complained of pain in the tongue.
(a) Give six causes of the general appearance.
(b) What is the diagnosis?
(c) To what is the pain due?

117

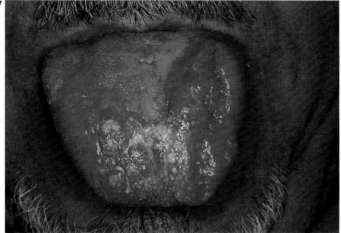

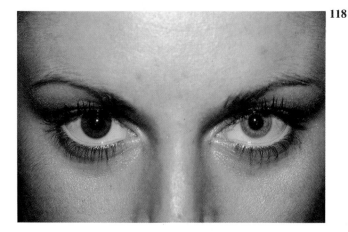

118 A woman complained of recurrent red eyes.
(a) What is the significance of the physical sign?
(b) What is the diagnosis?
(c) What may happen in middle-age?

119 A 10-year-old Nigerian Yoruba boy suffered from weight loss and a chronic cough.
(a) What diagnosis should be made from the appearance in the eye?
(b) What investigations would you perform?
(c) What other cutaneous allergic manifestations can occur in this condition?

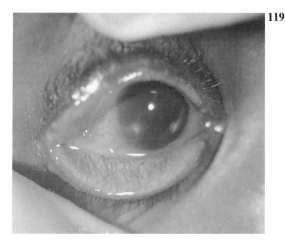

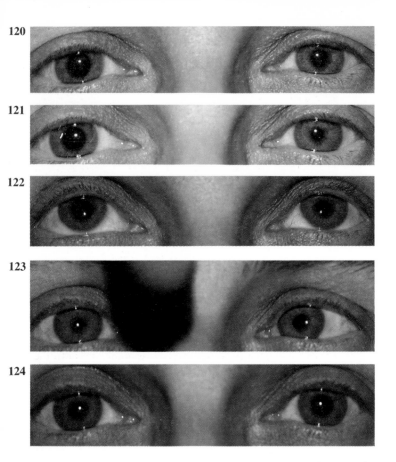

120–124 A young man presented with absent ankle jerks and a unilateral regular dilated pupil (**120**) which showed no change after exposure to light (**121**). He complained of sudden onset of blurred vision and noted a large pupil on the right; accommodation (**122**) produced constriction so that it was smaller than its fellow (**123**) and remained tonically contracted (**124**).

(a) Give four causes of a regular dilated pupil not reacting to light.
(b) What is the diagnosis?
(c) What is the differential diagnosis?
(d) Give three causes of small, irregular pupils.

125 An epileptic Asian woman presented with a waddling gait and proximal muscle weakness.
(a) What is the diagnosis?
(b) How may climate, custom, diet and therapy explain the X-ray appearances?

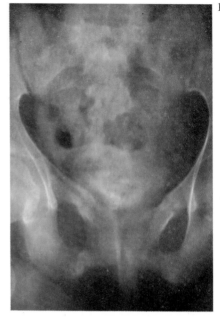

126 A heavy smoker complained of left chest pain radiating down the arm. Electrocardiography showed non-specific ST wave changes; a photograph was taken one day later.
(a) What is the diagnosis?
(b) How could it have been made earlier?
(c) What are the commonest sites?

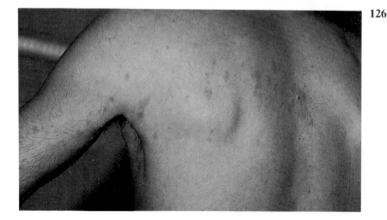

127

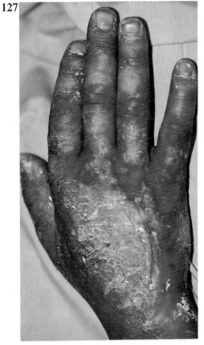

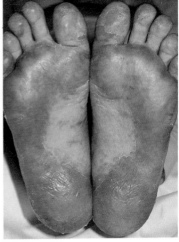

127–129 After a sore throat, blisters developed in the mouth of this patient with a rash on the hands, feet and scrotum.
(a) What is the diagnosis?
(b) How long had he been ill?
(c) Give five associated diseases.

129

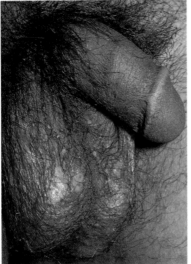

130 A 45-year-old man complained of tightness of the collar and shortness of breath.
(a) What is the physical sign?
(b) In which direction will the blood flow in the veins on the upper thorax?
(c) What is the diagnosis?
(d) What is the commonest cause for this condition?

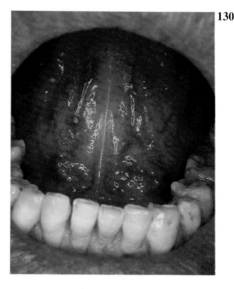

131 A 40-year-old civil engineer complained of impotence and night sweats.
(a) Give five neurological signs in this condition.
(b) What appearances are seen in the hands?
(c) What might be seen in the palms?
(d) What is the diagnosis?
(e) What causes the impotence?
(f) What causes the night sweats?

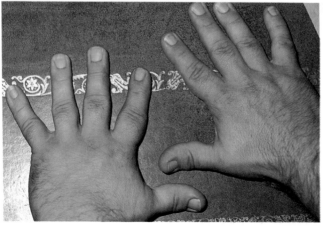

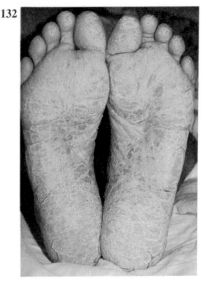

132 The patient complained of dysphagia for solids but not liquids.
(a) What investigation is appropriate and why?
(b) What other causes are associated with this physical sign?

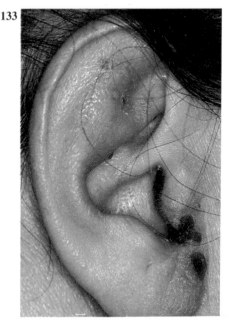

133 A patient, with normal eardrum, one day after onset of earache.
(a) What will sensory testing of the head show?
(b) What area is affected?
(c) What is the diagnosis?

134 A 50-year-old man, four days after operation for an inguinal hernia, developed a high fever followed by a rash.
(a) What is the diagnosis?
(b) What is the most common manifestation of this virus in this age group?
(c) Give four complications of this condition.

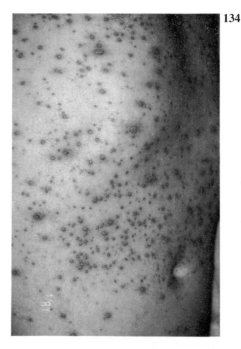

135 (a) What is the diagnosis?
(b) What is the deformity?
(c) To what is it due?

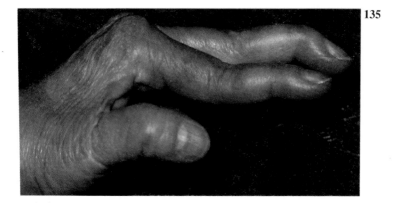

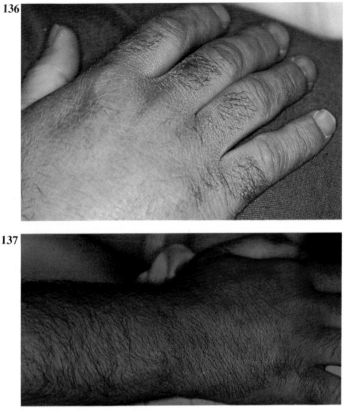

136, 137 A middle-aged man presents with cramps and constipation; there is a change in hair growth in his hand over a five-month period.
(a) Why may this have occurred?
(b) What is the diagnosis?

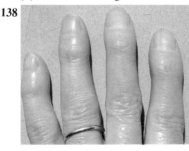

138 A woman presents with pain in the finger joints.
(a) Give two causes of this appearance and one confirmatory sign.
(b) What is the diagnosis?

139 An introspective man presented with recurrent shooting pains in the buttocks.
(a) What is the diagnosis?
(b) What is the differential diagnosis?
(c) Give three complications of this condition.

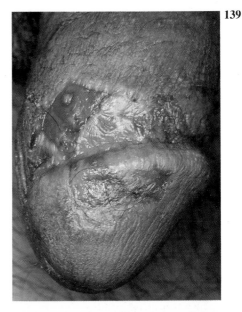

140 The topographic distribution of a rash may be helpful diagnostically; this man complained of a sore left nipple.
(a) Give four conditions where the presence or absence of a rash in the axilla may be helpful.
(b) What is distinctive about this particular rash?

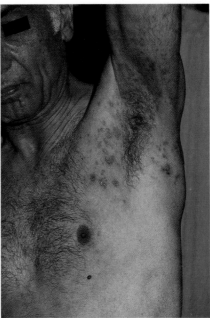

141

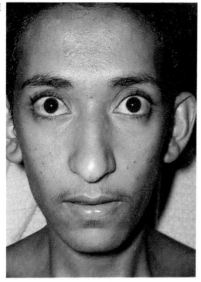

141 The presenting complaint was a poor golf swing with increasing shoulder weakness.
(a) What physical signs are seen?
(b) What eye signs may be found?
(c) What is the diagnosis?
(d) What other associated diseases could be present?

142 A woman complained of poor circulation aggravated by cold weather.
(a) What is the diagnosis?
(b) Give four secondary causes of this appearance.

142

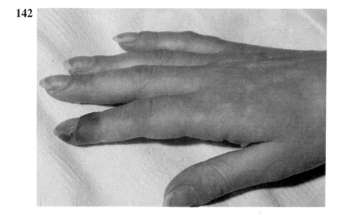

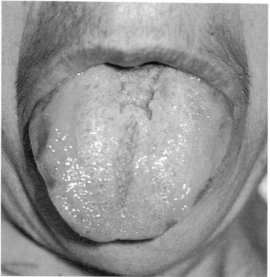

143 A 50-year-old patient complained of tingling of the hands at night. Give three possible reasons for this presentation.

144 A 32-year-old male presented with infertility.
(a) What is the diagnosis?
(b) Which hormone would you assay?
(c) Give six causes for normal elevation of this hormone.
(d) Give six causes for abnormal elevation of this hormone.

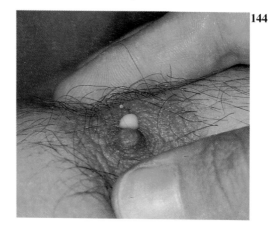

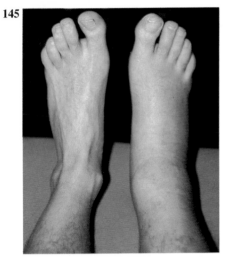

145 During a hiking trip a 35-year-old male complained of severe pain in the right foot preventing sleep. No fracture was seen on X-ray.
(a) What is the diagnosis?
(b) Why was the X-ray performed?
(c) What may have predisposed to the problem?

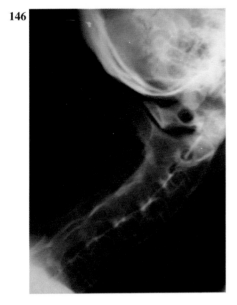

146 This patient's sister had longstanding granulomatous colitis.
(a) What is the diagnosis?
(b) What had they in common?
(c) What does his X-ray show?
(d) Give three associated non-articular complications of this condition.

147 A 49-year-old woman complained of pain in her right hand.
(a) What can be seen?
(b) What is the cause?
(c) What is the diagnosis?

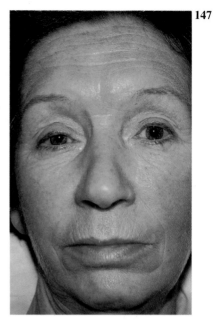

148 An 11-year-old girl noted stiffness and changes in the left hand.
(a) What is the diagnosis?
(b) What is the prognosis?

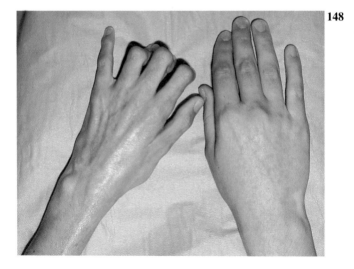

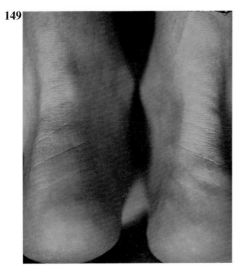

149 This patient's father had a myocardial infarction at the age of 35.
(a) What investigation is indicated?
(b) What other signs may be seen?

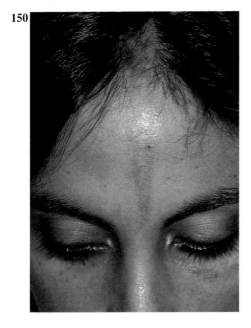

150 A young woman consults you worried that she is going to lose her hair.
(a) What is the diagnosis?
(b) Can you reassure her about it?
(c) What else may be affected?

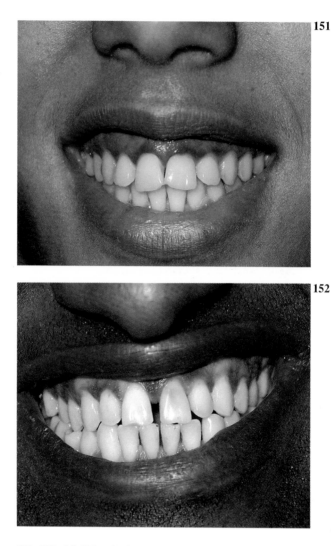

151, 152 (a) What is the diagnosis?
(b) Give three causes of the physical sign shown.

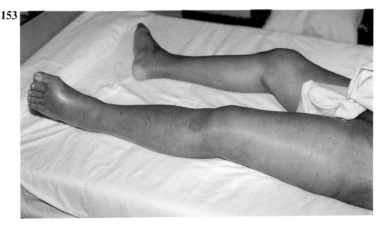

153 A 65-year-old male presented with weight loss, no physical signs and three weeks later developed this picture.
(a) What is the cause of the appearance?
(b) What is the diagnosis?
(c) What is the underlying problem?

154 (a) What is the diagnosis?
(b) Give four differential diagnoses.
(c) Give three associated diseases.
(d) Give two associated physical signs.
(e) Give one typical sign seen here.

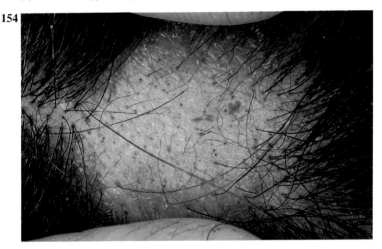

155 At 13.20 in the morning medical outpatient clinic, a receptionist had difficulty with an aggressive patient complaining of delay.

(a) Which clinic was running late?

(b) What was the problem?

(c) What other mechanism may be incriminated at this time of day?

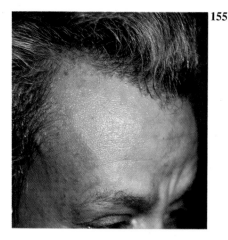

156 A 55-year-old man with diabetes presented with loss of libido and painful joints.

(a) What is the diagnosis?

(b) What changes are present in the skin (the left hand is a control)?

(c) What may be seen on X-ray of the joints?

(d) In what other conditions does the X-ray change occur?

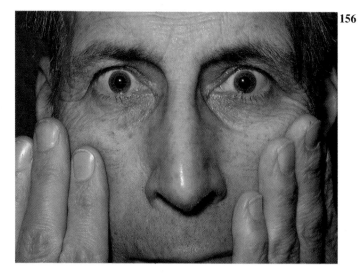

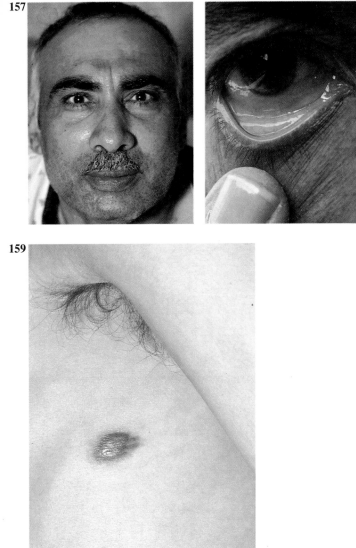

157–160 Three photographs have the fourth in common: (**157**) a man complaining of stiffness and slowness; (**158**) a man complaining of itching; (**159**) a man complaining of a rash; (**160**) a man with marks on his hand.
(a) What does each picture show?
(b) What is the link?

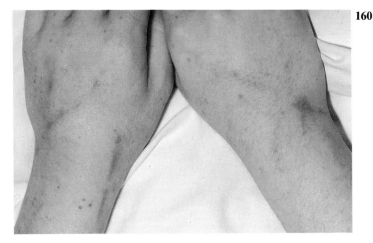

161 A 14-year-old girl presented with fever and abdominal colic.
(a) What is the diagnosis?
(b) Give four clinical features of this condition.
(c) Give four precipitating factors.

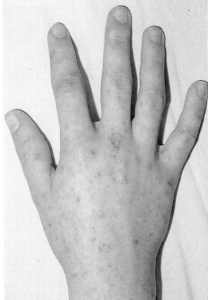

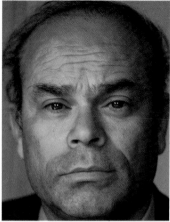

162 This patient complained of lack of drive (loss of ambition), tingling hands and hair loss on the dorsum of the hands.
(a) What is the diagnosis?
(b) Give four skin changes that can occur in this condition.
(c) Give three causes of the paraesthesiae.

163, 164 A 30-year-old man complained of nausea on waking in the morning.
(a) What is the diagnosis?
(b) Give four conditions associated with this appearance.
(c) Give four associated physical signs.

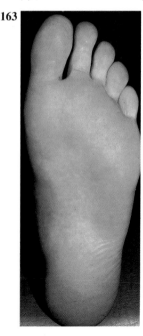

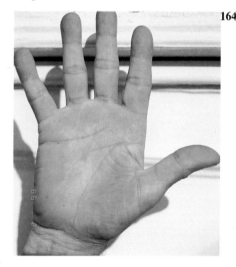

165 This is a classic facies.
(a) What is the diagnosis?
(b) Give three physical signs.
(c) Give five ocular manifestations.
(d) Give five atypical presentations of this condition.

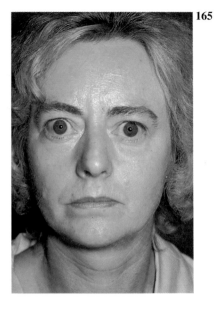

166 A child fails to gain weight and has loose stools.
(a) What physical sign is seen?
(b) What is the diagnosis?
(c) What is the cause?

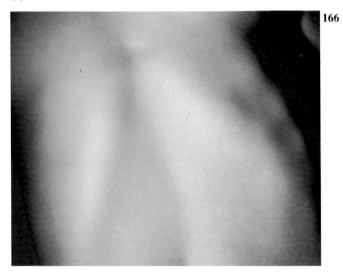

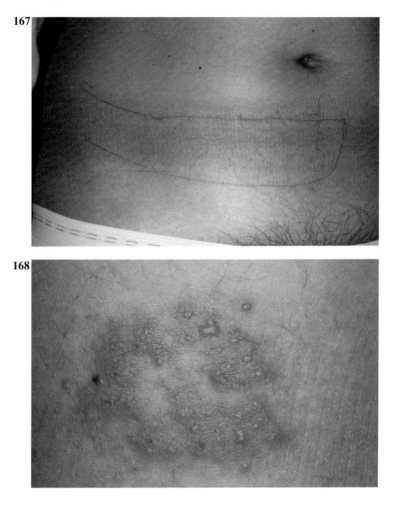

167, 168 A 20-year-old man has had right iliac fossa pain and tenderness for 24 hours; a rash is seen in the loin (**168**).
(a) What is the diagnosis?
(b) What physical signs can be found (**167**)?
(c) What physical signs might be seen 24 hours later?

169–171 A woman with pneumonia developed severe abdominal pain, aggravated by straining/coughing.

(a) What has caused the chest appearance (**169**)?

(b) What has caused the abdominal appearance (**170**)?

(c) Give five complications of coughing.

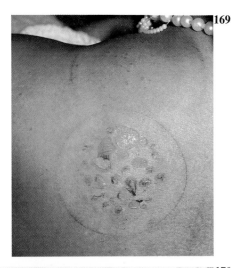

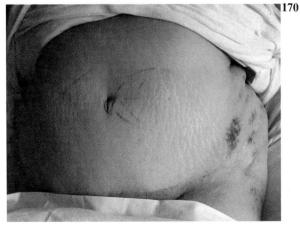

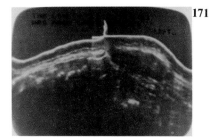

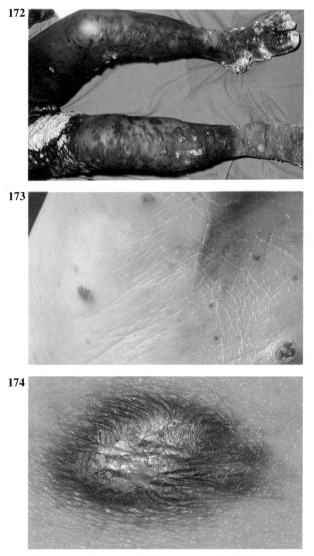

172–174 A Nigerian (**172**), an Israeli (**173**), and an American (**174**) presented with three variations of a condition, usually of short, medium or long-time span.
(a) What is the diagnosis?
(b) What are the types?
(c) Which is associated with a sexually transmitted disease?

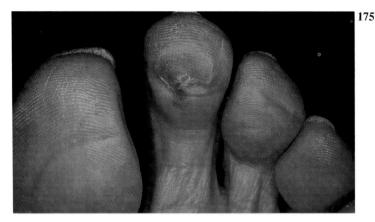

175 An English schoolboy presented with burning toes in winter.
(a) What is the diagnosis?
(b) Give three manifestations of this type of injury.

176 A Nigerian boy presented with pain in the bones.
(a) Why is he anaemic?
(b) What does the X-ray show?
(c) What is a likely organism?

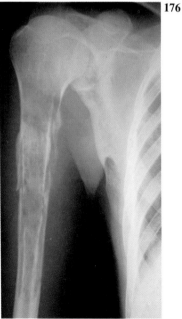

177

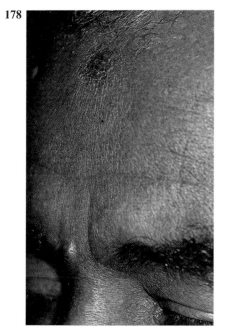

177 This patient complained of pains in the joint and ulceration on the foot.
(a) To what is the appearance due?
(b) How may this be prevented?

178

178 What is the significance of the physical sign seen?

179 A 35-year-old woman presented with constipation and a haemoglobin of 9.0 g/dl.
(a) What is the diagnosis?
(b) Give four possible reasons for her anaemia.

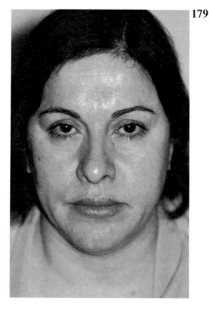

180 (a) What is the diagnosis?
(b) Give two causes of this condition that may affect the upper limb.
(c) Give three causes that may affect the lower limb.

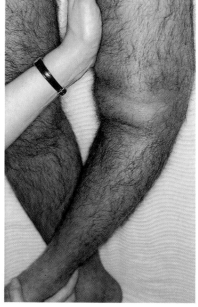

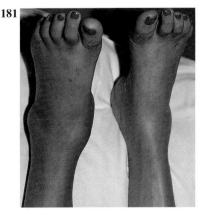

181 This 45-year-old insulin-dependent diabetic slipped on the kerb twisting her ankle, noting minor discomfort at the time, two months before this picture was taken.
(a) What is the diagnosis?
(b) Which other signs may be found?
(c) What is the significance of the dilated veins?
(d) What will the X-ray show?
(e) Give three other causes of this condition.

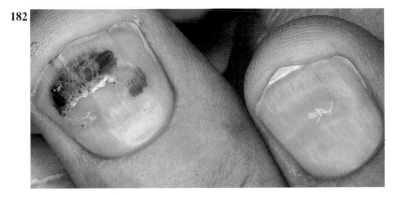

182 A man recovered from severe Stevens–Johnson syndrome, complicating erythema multiforme and a collagen disease. What facts about the history can be deduced from examination of his nails?

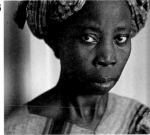

183 A Yoruba woman complained of stiffness and difficulty in eating.
(a) What is the diagnosis?
(b) Which two conditions may produce this physical sign?
(c) What are the classic features of this problem?

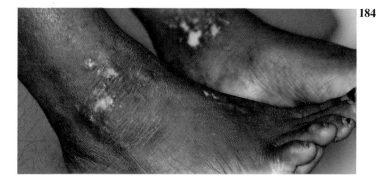

184 A Sudanese woman complained of itchy ankles.
(a) What is the diagnosis?
(b) Give four causes of depigmentation or hypopigmentation in a dark skin.
(c) Give an important differential diagnosis.

185 A 50-year-old man with pain in the hip developed an iron deficiency anaemia.
(a) What advice would you give him?
(b) Give several causes of similar appearances.
(c) What is the diagnosis?

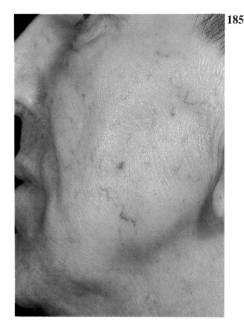

186 This young man was embarrassed if asked to shake hands during cold weather.
(a) Give two causes of this sign.
(b) Give two physical signs of this condition.

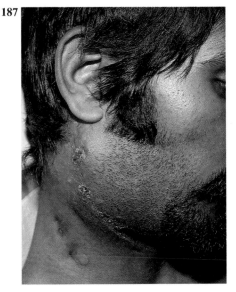

187 A farm worker presented with sore red eyes.
(a) What is the neck lesion?
(b) What is the eye lesion?
(c) What is the organism?
(d) What other sites may be affected?

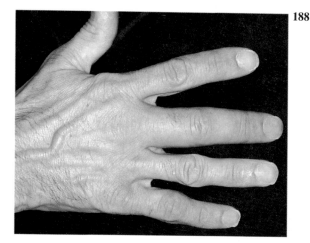

188 This patient presented with a mildly painful stiff finger.
(a) What is the diagnosis?
(b) What causes this appearance in short-term and long-term swelling?

189 A young man presented with recurrent headache.
(a) What is the appearance?
(b) Give possible causes of this physical sign.

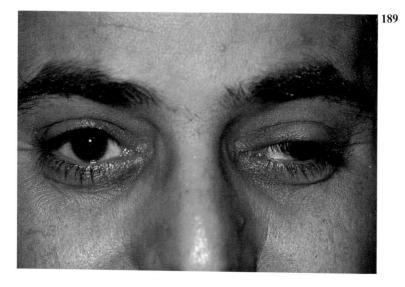

190

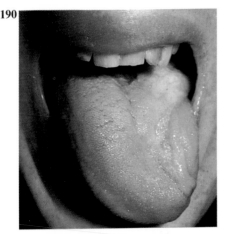

190 A Chinese waiter complained of a left-sided ptosis.
(a) What nerve(s) are affected?
(b) What is the site of the lesion?
(c) What is the likely diagnosis?

191

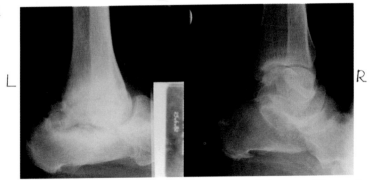

191 A woman presented with insulin-dependent diabetes mellitus and a hemiplegia.
(a) On which side is the hemiplegia?
(b) What is the cause of this appearance?

192

192 (a) How fast may this nail grow?
(b) Give several associated conditions.

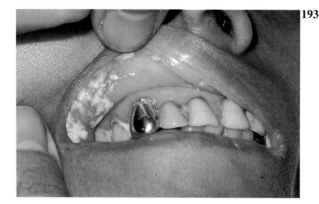

193 An air steward complained of dysphagia.
(a) What single fact in the social history is vital and what blood test is indicated?
(b) What other oral manifestations may occur in this condition?
(c) What is the differential diagnosis?

194 An apathetic irritable child presented with diarrhoea and a pot belly.
(a) What is the diagnosis?
(b) What is the significance of the abdominal distention and diarrhoea?
(c) Give four physical signs.
(d) What investigations should be carried out?

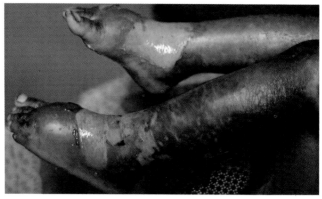

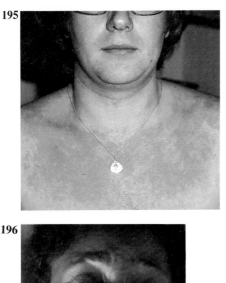

195 (a) Which three substances might be found in this man's urine?
(b) Suggest other causes of face flushing.

196 This patient shows a smile that does not reach the eyes.
(a) What is the diagnosis?
(b) What could cause this appearance?

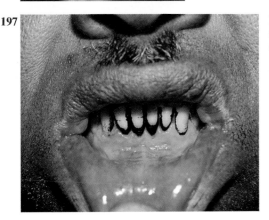

197 (a) What is the cause of this appearance?
(b) Of what is the patient at risk?

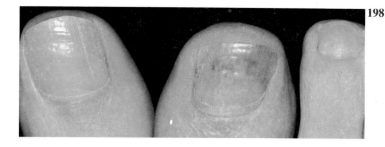

198

198, 199 A 35-year-old man presented with low back pain.
(a) What is the diagnosis?
(b) What other sites should be examined?
(c) What other causes may there be?

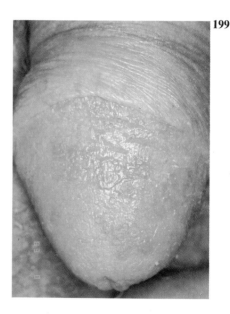

199

200 A bedouin Arab complained of fever and a lump in his neck.
(a) What could cause the lateral upper neck swelling?
(b) What is the most likely diagnosis?

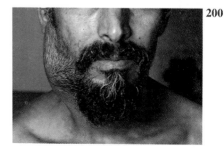

200

201

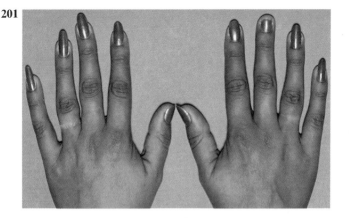

201 Why would this woman complain of increasing lethargy for six months before she consulted you, or why might a similar woman complain of increasing lethargy six months after completing her treatment?

202

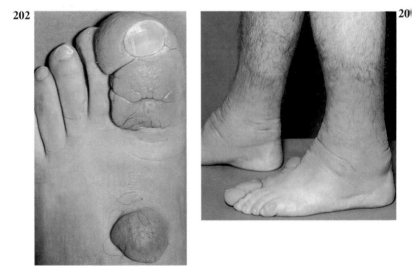

203

202, 203 A 40-year-old man presented with constipation, weight gain and double vision six months after therapy.
(a) What was the therapy?
(b) Why should his shoe size change?
(c) Why did he complain of diplopia?

204, 205 Each man, with facial weakness, has difficulty in eating and uses a hand on the mouth to assist. Responding to 'show me your teeth' and 'screw up your eyes'.

(a) What are the two diagnoses?

(b) What muscles are supported by the hand in each case during eating?

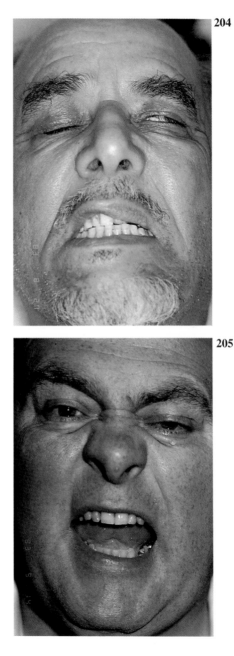

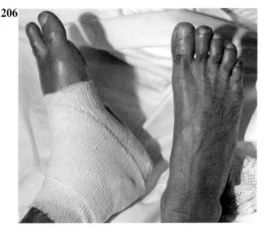

206 This diabetic suffered from nocturnal diarrhoea.
(a) What findings in his foot are related to the cause of the diarrhoea?
(b) How do they aggravate diabetic foot complications?
(c) What is the diagnosis?
(d) What other general features of this condition are there?

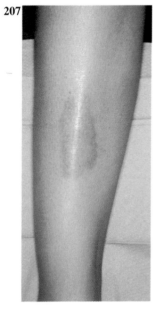

207 A young woman has a chronic skin lesion on the legs.
(a) What is the diagnosis?
(b) What may be found in the urine?
(c) What other skin conditions may be found in her or her family?

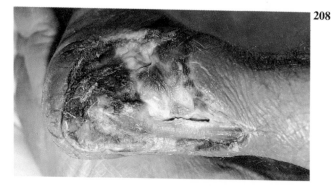

208 Two weeks earlier, this diabetic's foot appeared normal but in spite of ampicillin, this foot infection developed.
(a) What has been overlooked?
(b) What should have been prescribed?
(c) Why is a sense of smell important?

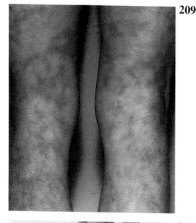

209 (a) Give three causes of this appearance.
(b) Give two possible diagnoses.

210 This girl has weight loss, dysphagia and weakness.
(a) What is the diagnosis?
(b) What is seen on the hands?
(c) What may be seen on the face?

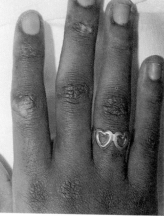

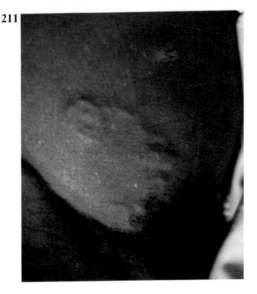

211 (a) What is the diagnosis in this African farmer?
(b) What may be seen on the chest X-ray?

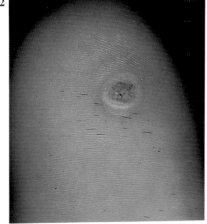

212 (a) What group of viruses causes this condition?
(b) What is the significance of the black dots?
(c) Give three situations of increased frequency of these lesions.

213 A three-year-old Nigerian complained of vomiting, headache and fever.

(a) What is a likely cause for the symptoms?

(b) What is a likely cause in this child?

(c) What complication may have occurred?

(d) What is the diagnosis?

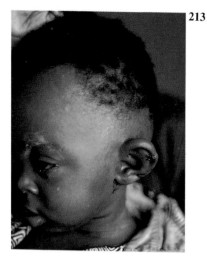

213

214 (a) What other sites would you examine, having found this physical sign?

(b) What is seen in the elbow?

(c) Give five differential diagnoses.

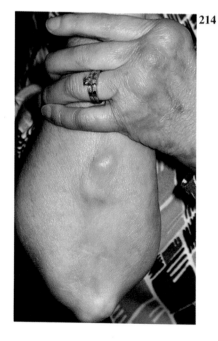

214

215

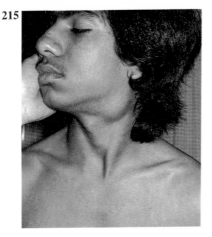

215 A 17-year-old male presented with recent febrile illness and sore throat.
(a) Give four possible diagnoses.
(b) What is the actual diagnosis?

216 (a) Note three physical changes and comment on each.
(b) Which is the odd one out and to what may it be due?
(c) What is the diagnosis?

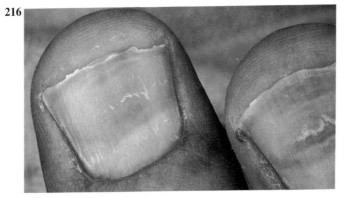

216

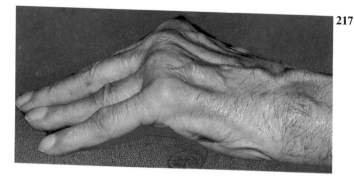

217 A 55-year-old male electrician suffered a severe electric shock at work.
(a) What is the diagnosis?
(b) What has happened?
(c) What may examination of the feet and tongue show?

ANSWERS

1 (a) A red rash over the knuckles and nail beds with thinning of the skin which in the caucasian is pink with pink induration of the nail beds, and in the coloured skin shows up as a dark rash with thinning over the knuckles and at the nail beds; heliotrope rash around the eyes, associated with periorbital oedema; easy bruising after gripping of the skin.
(b) A search for occult tumours — carcinoma and lymphoma, particularly in individuals over the age of 40 where the incidence is increased fivefold; electromyography (EMG) — characteristic changes differentiate it from a myopathy; serum creatinine phosphokinase (CPK) and aldolase are usually elevated.
(c) Polymyositis; collagen disease and neoplasia.

2 (a) Clubbing: a high proportion exhibit this sign in cystic fibrosis with its lung suppuration. Other causes include cyanotic congenital heart disease, bacterial endocarditis and fibrosing alveolitis. Gastroenterological associated diseases include Crohn's disease, biliary cirrhosis and malabsorption syndromes.
(b) Thyroid acropachy; clubbing may develop 6 months after thyrotoxicosis is treated.
(c) Thyroid acropachy, where pains occur in the long bones, X-ray shows periosteal new bone formation, and spicules of bone grow perpendicularly; hypertrophic pulmonary osteoarthropathy is also associated with clubbing, pains in the long bones and periosteal reactions, and bone is laid down longitudinally subperiosteally.

3 (a) Bony overgrowth on the dorsolateral aspect of the terminal interphalangeal (IP) joint in osteoarthrosis — Heberden's nodes.
(b) Terminal IP joint — Heberden's nodes; proximal IP joint — Bouchard's nodes; carpometacarpal joint of the thumbs — often shown by loss of joint space (cartilage) on X-ray.

4 (a) Dystrophia myotonica. Physical signs show a female with bilateral ptosis and wasting of the facial muscles.
(b) Congenital, tabetic, myopathic/myasthenic, functional.
(c) Aspiration pneumonia secondary to difficulty in swallowing due to pharyngeal and diaphragmatic involvement, plus the risk of cardiac conduction defects.
(d) Increased stiffness of muscles (myotonia), worse in cold temperatures.

5 (a) Scarlet fever. A red maculopapular rash is present, sparing the perioral and periorbital areas. There is no scleral injection. The throat was sore and grew a streptococcus.
(b) Includes erythema multiforme, streptococcal scarlet fever, leptospirosis, toxic shock syndrome (enquire about tampon (vaginal) use). Association of menstruation and fever makes the diagnosis of toxic shock syndrome more likely than scarlet fever, although it may be part of the syndrome of staphylococcal scarlet fever, the rash which may be associated with streptococcal infections of the upper respiratory tract, wound infection or impetigo. It presents with pyrexia, headache, vomiting and a punctate erythematous rash, most probably a sensitivity reaction, which peels as it fades. The tongue may show a characteristic 'strawberry' appearance.

6 (a) Oestrogens for carcinoma of the prostate or spironolactone for ascites.
(b) Bilateral well-marked gynaecomastia; a right upper paramedian scar; the abdomen is distended, an umbilical hernia contains fluid; bruising at the costal margin and above the symphysis. The appearances are those of ascites with a bleeding diathesis. Spider naevi are just discernible at the neck. Cirrhosis of the liver can be inferred.

7 (a) Erythrocyte sedimentation rate (ESR).
(b) Would include polymyalgia rheumatica, and an ESR would point towards this.
(c) Herpes zoster. The rash affects the distribution of the second cervical dermatome, sparing the cheek, the tragus and the anterior part of the pinna which is enervated by the third branch of the Vth nerve. There is some crusting where vesicles have ruptured affecting the upper part of the pinna, the anterior part of the lobe and along the jawline, outlining the second cervical dermatome. The crusting can be seen inside the hairline and her headache was the neuralgic pain that occurs before the appearance of the rash.
(d) A plaque of disseminated sclerosis in the late acute stage; polyneuritis or transverse myelitis; extradural cord compression by metastases. Paralysis will be *below* the level of the herpetic eruption.

8 (a) Widening at the wrist and immediately above the ankle joint is characteristic of rickets and caused by an excess of uncalcified osteoid.
(b) Nutritional, due to poor intake or synthesis in the skin, malabsorption, renal disease and anticonvulsant therapy.
(c) In the elderly and immigrants the intake of vitamin D in the food may be poor, food constituents may bind calcium and sunlight may be unavailable or screened from the skin by clothes or pigmentation; bone pain is often the presenting feature.
(d) Rickets, hand and foot.

9 (a) Sickle cell anaemia — he suffers from fever, abdominal pain and ischaemic necrosis of both upper femora and humeri with pathological fractures.
(b) Avoid anoxia during induction, for he has sickle cell bone disease with infarction and a residual short digit secondary to dactylitis 6 years previously. This disease characteristically involves the digits of the fingers and toes, and may lead to ischaemic necrosis and shortening of the digit, with pain as a presenting feature.
(c) Salmonellae, causing secondary infection in the bone.

10 (a) The feet exhibit signs of ischaemia, and four fingers have been lost. The skin of the feet is dry and atrophic, no hairs are visible on the toes, the nails are dystrophic and deformed — all characteristics of the poor blood supply. There is also gangrene of the right third toe and the left great toe is missing.
(b) Buerger's disease (thromboangiitis obliterans).

11 (a) The left hand is normal, but oedema of the right hand is affecting the dorsum of the palm and fingers with loss of the skinfolds. This may be related to dactylitis with bone cysts as in sarcoidosis. As the swelling affects the hand and arm, disuse related to hemiplegia is more likely although venous thrombosis, lymphatic obstruction or surgical lymphatic ablation cannot be excluded.
(b) Cerebral haemorrhage and a hemiplegia.

12 (a) Urine test for sugar.
(b) The brown distal band (secondary to telangiectasia) and white or pale pink area suggest non-insulin-dependent diabetes mellitus, cirrhosis of the liver or congestive cardiac failure and in association with increasing age.

13 (a) At the base of the fingernail there is a red area which did not blanch on pressure; a similar appearance is seen on the skin of the lower limb on which the finger rests. There was also fever, arthralgia, foot drop and patchy lung shadowing.

(b) It is characteristic of a vasculitis in an immune complex disease; the physical sign is non-specific in the spectrum of this multisystem disorder, but it may occur in rheumatoid arthritis, systemic lupus erythematosus (SLE), immune complex disease such as Henoch–Schönlein's purpura. In rheumatoid arthritis it is often associated with nodule formation and skin ulceration.

(c) Polyarteritis nodosa on biopsy. She was hepatitis B antigen-negative.

(d) Viral haemorrhagic fevers.

14 (a) Smallpox primary immunisation scar — smallpox was eradicated in 1980; BCG immunisation against tuberculosis, now ulcerating. The regional lymph glands are enlarged and can be seen in the anterior triangle of the neck. The condition will resolve, and this can be speeded by use of isoniazid.

(b) BCG ulcer and lymphadenopathy.

15, 16 (a) Poor technique; upper brain stem lesions (there is inability to converge the eyes and therefore loss of pupillary reaction); Parkinson's disease (there is also failure of convergence). Compare these pictures with **120–124**.

(b) Diphtheria.

17 (a) The changes are those of ridging; longitudinal ridges are seen more frequently in middle and old age. There is minor beading of the ridges down the left side of the thumb nail, most frequently seen in rheumatoid arthritis.

(b) There is a transverse depression across the middle of the nail in the junction of the middle and proximal thirds above the lunula, first described by Guillaume Beau in 1840. There is disturbance of nail growth with a systemic upset; since the nail grows at the rate of ½–1 mm/day, an illness probably occurred about 6 weeks earlier.

18–21 (a) Proptosis of the eyeball not associated with lid retraction and only apparent on viewing from above with the lid raised; diplopia was also present.

(b) Orbital tumour; orbital pseudotumour; endocrine exophthalmos; carotico-cavernous fistula.

(c) Cavernous fistula as there is no conjunctival injection.

(d) Orbital pseudotumour, demonstrated by CT scan.

22 (a) Kayser–Fleischer ring — brown pigment deposited at the limbus seen in hepatolenticular degeneration (Wilson's disease).

(b) The abdomen may show hepatosplenomegaly, as he has portal hypertension and varices; the arms show tremor and rigidity.

23 (a) Arcus cornealis, due to deposition of lipids, at the junction of the cornea and sclera on Descemet's membrane; it is present in many people over 50 years of age and may be partial or complete.

(b) Xanthomata may be present on the skin or in tendon, pointing to a disorder (rare) of lipid metabolism; these should be looked for in young people particularly, as relevant to future management.

24 (a) Lymph gland enlargement associated with the lymphangitis seen as a red streak.

(b) Open pulmonary tuberculosis.

(c) Reaction to the injection of old tuberculin (5 TU) — the Mantoux test — can be subdivided into those with induration smaller than 10 mm and those of larger size due to infection with *Mycobacterium tuberculosis*. In Denmark and North America less than 10 per cent will show non-specific reactions, whereas in Asia and India the proportion may rise to 80 per cent. Young persons who are strongly positive tuberculin reactors should receive chemoprophylaxis. Tuberculosis contacts may require BCG, if Mantoux negative.

25 (a) Diplopia is present, the eye is pushed outwards and downwards; there is a IIIrd nerve palsy, proptosis with a thrill over the medial end of the left eyebrow, and the mass pulsates.
(b) Auscultation will demonstrate the bruit, which is audible both to the examiner and the patient; it can be suppressed by compressing the carotid artery on the left side.
(c) There is unilateral pulsating exophthalmos with oedema of both eyelids, injection of the conjunctivae and left-sided papilloedema. The injection in the right eye is caused by the communication through the circular sinus to the opposite cavernous sinus.
(d) Secondary to a ruptured aneurysm or fracture of the skull, blood drains anteriorly via the ophthalmic veins to the face, leading to oedema of the muscles and external ocular muscle paralysis. The fistulae are more common in disorders of supporting tissues.
(e) Caroticocavernous fistula.

26–29 (a) Congenital, present from birth; tabetic, pupillary changes; myasthenic, comes on with fatigue; myopathic, constant. Generally, frontalis overreaction will be present in the first two and absent in the second two (**29**).
(b) The inability to close the eyes and cover the eyelashes due to weakness of the orbicularis oculi, and myasthenic snarl are apparent. There is weakness of the corners of the mouth so that the teeth cannot be shown easily, and the jaw is weak so that the teeth cannot be clenched. These appearances are typical of myasthenia gravis. **27–29** demonstrate fatigue coming on with prolonged upward gaze; ptosis which becomes bilateral, with weakness of abduction of the left eye, is almost complete with minimal reaction of the frontalis, and would be instantly relieved by edrophonium injection.

30 (a) Gangrene of the tip of the ring finger with a line of demarcation just distal to the terminal interphalangeal joint. Ischaemic changes are visible on the ulnar border of the middle finger. The nails are normal, with no Beau's lines, inferring that this is an acute occlusion of a small vessel affecting the tips of the fingers.
(b) Ergotism, Raynaud's phenomenon, cervical rib with emboli, or a multisystem disease with vasculitis such as lupus erythematosus (LE).

31 (a) Scleroderma: there is reabsorption of the terminal phalanx of both index fingers, the skin is taut and hard, with the changes of chronic Raynaud's phenomenon in both hands.
(b) The lung — lower lobe fibrosis and crackles on auscultation; the gut — oesophageal involvement, dysphagia and pneumatosis cystoides intestinalis; the kidney — hypertension, proteinuria and renal failure; the joints — polyarthralgia in 25 per cent, with joint stiffness and limitation of movement.

32 (a) Wasting of the first dorsal interossei on both sides is seen as a depression in the tissues between the thumb and index finger, related in this man to a peripheral neuropathy and diabetes mellitus. The nerve supply of the first dorsal interosseus is from the ulnar nerve.
(b) Ptosis and Horner's syndrome secondary to interference with the sympathetic outflow at T1 (the segmental nerve supply of the small muscles of the hand).

33 (a) Iron deficiency. A spoon-shaped depression of the nail plate is seen here, which could contain a drop of water, and proximally is a transverse line due to disturbance of growth — Beau's line. Some 18 per cent of those suffering from iron deficiency demonstrate brittle, spoon-shaped flattening of the nails.
(b) Commonly glossitis — 40 per cent — and sometimes difficulties with swallowing and a postcricoid web. In the female the commonest cause is bleeding due to menorrhagia. This appearance is not specific for iron deficiency and may occur in any systemic upset over a period of time when there will be disturbance of nail growth; in infants and small children it is a normal phase of growth.
(c) Koilonychia, which may be developmental, associated with iron deficiency, due to a local cause such as Raynaud's phenomenon, and occasionally found in diabetics.

34 (a) Bouchard's nodes in osteoarthritis.
(b) Bony and cartilagenous enlargement in interphalangeal joints. Feel the hand, and unlike joint swelling this is localised to the dorsal and dorsomedial aspects, and may be associated with flexion and lateral deviation of the distal phalanx. The terminal interphalangeal joint swelling is Heberden's node, and the proximal interphalangeal joint Bouchard's node — usually single, occasionally multiple, more common in women than in men.
(c) Small gelatinous cysts may develop adjacent to these nodes.

35 (a) Beading of the nail in rheumatoid arthritis. The nail shows longitudinal ridging and beading, is more common in old age than youth and in the over-30s, and in rheumatoid arthritis than in controls. The nailfold shows vasculitis.
(b) Seropositive rheumatoid arthritis associated with gross subcutaneous nodules.

36 (a) The left hand, as the girl has a hemiplegia and is able to manicure the fingernails of the paralysed hand with the good hand.
(b) The leg in particular showed oedema; atrophy and blotchiness of the cool skin with slight wasting and oedema; mild wasting; coolness.
(c) Disuse osteoporosis.

37 (a) Dilated veins on the chest.
(b) Mediastinal obstruction, associated with a plethoric face, oedema of the head and neck, distention of the neck and sublingual veins, stridor and oedema of the arms. Direction of flow is downwards to bypass the superior vena caval block.

38 (a) Congenital 'fissured' scrotal (large) tongue.
(b) Large tongues occur in the Melkersson–Rosenthal syndrome with thick lips — granulomatous cheilitis — recurrent facial palsy, differential diagnosis being from sarcoid and Crohn's disease; acromegaly with indentation of the tongue produced by teeth; Down's syndrome (a large folded tongue); hypothyroidism — reversible.

39 (a) Dilated tortuous temporal artery, which may be tender or reddened; note that this may be a normal variant.
(b) Erythrocyte sedimentation rate (ESR) may be elevated beyond 35 mm in the first hour, although temporal arteritis may occur with a low ESR.
(c) Arteritis; biopsy may be negative due to the patchy nature of the lesion.
(d) Polymyalgia rheumatica, on the clinical picture.

40 (a) Yellow palms of carotenaemia and hypothyroidism; the sclerae remain white, differentiating it from jaundice.
(b) An accumulation of betacarotene in the skin, due to a defect in the enzymatic conversion of vitamin A in hypothyroidism.

(c) A high dietary intake of vitamin A as carrots, mangoes or oranges — it is benign and clears on reducing intake; in association with hyperbetalipoproteinaemia; in treatment with betacarotene to combat solar sensitivity in erythropoietica protoporphyria.

41 (a) Lichen planus.
(b) The lacelike pattern of 'Wickham's striae' differentiates this from the coarser pattern of leukoplakia. If erosion occurs, gingivitis, aphthous ulceration and erythema multiforme may need to be excluded. Scraping of the white patches will reveal the redness of monilia.
(c) Wrist flexures where flat-topped violaceous pruritic papules are noted, also seen on the ankles and penis. The hair, which may show patchy alopecia. The nails, for dystrophy.
(d) By drugs such as anti-TB treatment, methyldopa, arsenicals; skin lesions can be related to sunlight.

42, 43 (a) An olecranon bursa which may be secondary to trauma or arise spontaneously.
(b) Closer examination (**43**) shows the white crystals of sodium urate showing through the skin.
(c) Gouty tophus.
(d) The helix and antihelix of the ear, the fingers, the dorsum of the joints, knees, feet, and the ulnar surface of the forearm; tophi must be differentiated from rheumatoid nodules — they appear in areas which tend to be cooler than the body core.

44 (a) Relapsing polychondritis.
(b) The eyes (redness); the ears ('felt-like' consistency); nasal deformity; tracheomalacia and tender costochondral junctions.
(c) Wegener's granulomatosis: necrotising vasculitis affecting nasal septum leads to collapse — 85 per cent will have renal disease and the urine should always be tested when this sign is seen. Congenital syphilis: deformity occurs in infancy and may be associated with frontal bossing secondary to osteoperiostitis (Parrot's nodes). Scars at the angles of the mouth (rhagades), notched incisors and corneal nebulae are secondary to interstitial keratitis.

45 (a) A pterygium, a sheaf of vessels growing across the cornea from the sclera, occurring in relation to severe climatic conditions and of no serious importance. It requires no treatment unless it encroaches on the visual axis, and is more common in coloured races. An early cataract.
(b) Diabetes mellitus; trauma; ionising radiation; dystrophia myotonica; hypocalcaemia; steroid therapy.

46–48 (a) ACTH-dependent Cushing's syndrome with diabetes mellitus, secondary to adrenocortical hyperplasia. Signs: **46** — hirsutes, mild facial mooning and livid striae of the forearm with thinness of the hair; **47** — the back pain due to vertebral collapse — kyphosis, and shoulder girdle muscle wasting due to protein catabolism; **48** — enlarged and demineralised pituitary fossa secondary to an ACTH-producing pituitary tumour.
(b) If adrenalectomy is performed pigmentation may occur due to continuing ACTH production by the pituitary tumour.

49 (a) Splinter haemorrhage of the nails is dubious physical evidence.

(b) Traditionally it is associated with bacterial endocarditis but is common in the general population and due to minor trauma, particularly in older age groups; also seen more frequently in rheumatoid arthritis; it may be associated with trichinosis.

(c) Rheumatoid arthritis — ridging and beading of the nail and a splinter is more common in this than in a control population, although no nailfold vasculitis is seen.

50, 51 (a) Linear naevus: a longitudinal band of pigmentation is present in the nail plate, probably related to a junctional naevus of the nail matrix with pigment overflowing into the nail.

(b) Yes. Junctional subungual naevi may become more pigmented in Addison's disease (hypoadrenocorticalism).

(c) Linear naevi may become malignant. In coloured skins pigmented streaks in the nail are commonly due to trauma.

52–54 (a) Recurrent relapsing polychondritis with softening and collapsing cartilagenous structures in the body.

(b) The pinna is red and swollen. The earlobe is spared as only the pinna contains cartilage — biopsy shows intense infiltration of cartilage which liquifies and the ear collapses like wet felt. The eye is inflamed due to scleritis as the globe has a similar structure to cartilage.

(c) A hoarse voice due to involvement of the larynx may be associated with stridor from tracheal ring softening; collapse of the nasal cartilage and tenderness of the costal cartilage may occur.

55, 56 (a) Ochronosis: the grey colour of the ear is caused by pigment in the cartilage which calcifies accounting for the stiff stonelike ear. The grey pigment may also be seen overlying tendons, joints and in the eye. Premature osteoarthritis occurs. Differentiate from the greyness of the skin in haemochromatosis which may also be associated with a seronegative large joint arthritis.

(b) It may darken as it oxidises overnight appearing grey/brown in colour. This pigment may produce colour changes on testing the urine with Benedict's solution and interfere with glucose oxidase reactions in dipstick tests for glycosuria.

57 Terminal brown arcs are found in renal failure, cirrhosis, diabetes, cardiac failure; linear bands may be related to trauma and are of no consequence; azure arcs confined to the lunula are seen in Wilson's disease (hepatolenticular degeneration); red arcs may be noted in cardiac failure; white nails are associated with hypoalbuminaemia.

58 (a) Functional ptosis. Slight ptosis of the left eyelid is associated with over-reaction of the frontalis, which is not on the same side as it should be if this were organic, but on the opposite side.

(b) Bilateral — myopathic, congenital or tabetic; unilateral — frontalis reaction is less likely in myopathies and should be on the same side as the ptosis; pupillary changes are seen in the IIIrd and sympathetic nerve lesions.

59 (a) An opposed thumb with a wasted thenar eminence.

(b) Abductor pollicis brevis.

(c) The median nerve and the first thoracic segment.

(d) Carpal tunnel syndrome.

(e) Acromegaly, hypothyroidism, pregnancy, the premenstrual period.

60, 61 (a) Tight skin and sausage-like fingers of scleroderma — differentiate from the fat finger of oedema in hemiplegia, myxoedema and increased soft tissues of acromegaly. Calcification is seen in the fingertip; calcinosis is associated with tuft resorption; vitiligo, usually associated with hyperpigmentation and telangiectasia.

(b) Linear atrophy-localised morphoea; no systemic manifestations, usually found as thickened skin or 'sabre-cut' atrophy (coup de sabre). CRST syndrome (calcinosis, Raynaud's phenomenon; sclerodactyly; telangiectasia), occasionally associated with exposure to polyvinylchloride (PVC). Progressive systemic sclerosis with multisystem involvement.

(c) Pulmonary—fibrosis and pulmonary hypertension; cardiac—fibrosis and conduction defects; renal—proteinuria, hypertension and renal failure; gut—oesophageal dysmotility; small joints—arthritis.

62 (a) Wasting of the first dorsal interosseus muscle.

(b) A small pupil on the right with partial ptosis — cervical sympathetic nerve lesion.

(c) T1 segment via the lower cords of the brachial plexus — 1st dorsal interosseus supplied by the ulnar nerve.

(d) Pancoast syndrome of carcinoma of the bronchus at the apex of the lung, involving small muscle wasting, weak medial wrist flexors, numb medial hand and Horner's syndrome.

63 (a) Dermatomyositis.

(b) Dermatomyositis: facial oedema and erythema, myalgia and proximal muscle weakness. Cushing's disease: facial mooning, oedema, plethora and proximal muscle weakness. Thyroid disease: thyrotoxic myopathy, thyroid facies — hypo-thyroidism with facial swelling and proximal myopathy. Myasthenia: eye changes of ptosis, and weakness on exertion on climbing stairs relieved by rest.

(c) Periorbital oedema; erythema, seen as a heliotrope rash but having a blue tint in coloured skin; reddened raised plaques over the extensor joint surfaces, dark in a coloured skin (collodion patches); telangiectasia, seen as reddened areas, dark in pigmented skin.

(d) Malignancy from the breast, thyroid or gut (in 10 per cent of dermatomyositis/polymyositis patients, more often in the older than younger age groups).

64 (a) Patchy limbal pigmentation.

(b) Argyria: grey sclera secondary to application of silver nitrate to the eyes, leading to a generalised dark grey pigmentation of the sclera. Kayser–Fleischer rings: a brown semicomplete or complete arc at the junction of the sclera, the limbus, deposited on Descemet's membrane on the inside of the cornea, usually with a narrow clear area adjacent to the limbus. Ochronosis: seen here as brown patchy pigmentation on the sclera near the limbus; also seen in the cartilage of the ear.

65–67 (a) A full volume pulse, tachycardia and an elevated jugular venous pressure — a high output failure. This is an extremely uncommon complication of Paget's disease, but may be due to secondary shunting of blood through a vascular area in polyostotic Paget's.

(b) In children, blood disease, sickle disease and thalassaemia; in adults, infection, syphilis, congenital Parrot's nodes and acromegaly; in the elderly, Paget's disease.

(c) Fractures, neurological sequelae from nerve compression and bone pains.

(d) The right leg is warmer, bowed and the bone has expanded.

(e) Locally — fracture, tumour, sarcoma, benign giant cell tumour, reparative granuloma. Generally — extramedullary haematopoiesis, cardiac failure secondary to high output state, deafness and narrowing of interosseus foraminae associated with muscular weakness.

(f) Increased density and expansion of the vertebral body.

68 (a) Ptosis; Horner's syndrome. The left lid cuts the pupil tangentially compared to the right.
(b) There is no pupillary constriction, no evidence of diminished sweating and no enophthalmos.
(c) A wasted left sternomastoid suggests spinal accessory involvement at the base of the skull, but a cough suggests a search for wasting of the small muscle of the hand in association with apical carcinoma. Dissociated sensory loss may be a feature from central cord lesions — look for burns on the hands.
(d) Tumour at the base of the skull.

69 (a) Gouty tophi: osteoarthritis affects the terminal interphalangeal joints, proximal interphalangeal joints and the index and middle finger may produce swellings of Bouchard's and Heberden's nodes, but there is reddening, erythema and peeling over these swellings and the white paste of urate shows through the skin.
(b) Uric acid calculi and renal failure.

70–73 (a) Nodule in the anterior part of the neck — recent appearance of a nodule represents a cysticercosis cyst (confirmed by X-ray of another nodule in the limb where it can be seen calcified).
(b) He is a vegetarian but the parasite exists in meat, so his cook may have contaminated the food.
(c) Showed 17 palpable subcutaneous nodules. X-ray of the forearm shows a calcified parasite *(arrow)*; CT scan shows an intracerebral cysticercus cyst — an area of increased attenuation surrounded by a ring of increased density. Biopsy of this nodule under polarised light shows the chitinous hooks. The tapeworm — *Taenia solium* — forms an encysted larva which is found in contaminated food from infected food handlers. The embryos, liberated by gastric juice, penetrate blood vessels, finally forming 1 cm diameter cysts. A common cause of epilepsy in South East Asia.

74 (a) Chondrocalcinosis of ear cartilage.
(b) Haemochromatosis; gout; pseudogout; Wilson's disease; hyperparathyroidism; degenerative joint disease; ochronosis, particularly the cartilage of joints and the pinna.
(c) Ochronosis.

75 (a) Dupuytren's contracture of the plantar fascia. Compared with the palmar type it is less of a problem — contractures do not occur; nodules, single or multiple, are not painful and sited in the non-weight-bearing instep; no thickening is seen over the interphalangeal toe.
(b) Contracture of the palmar fascia in 50 per cent of patients; fibrosis of the corpora cavernosa of the penis.

76, 77 A march fracture — there is a swelling over the anterior forefoot. Gout or pseudogout, although a first episode usually occurs in the great toe; forefoot pain and swelling may be the first sign precipitated after exercise and be confused with cellulitis; Morton's metatarsalgia — a plantar digital neuroma associated with pain between the third and fourth, and fourth and fifth spaces, increased on lateral pressure. In children, osteochondritis of the second metatarsal head.

78 (a) Dupuytren's contracture of the palmar fascia.
(b) Alcoholism, rather than cirrhosis; epilepsy; diabetes retinopathy trauma.

79 (a) Shiny nails.
(b) Lacquer; friction; to scratch, the distal third of the nail is rubbed against the skin with the hand in a semiclosed fist. Only a third of the nail has a high mirror finish; if lacquer all the nail is shiny.
(c) Bile — obstructive jaundice and pruritus; sugar — diabetes mellitus and pruritus.

80 (a) Erythema nodosum due to primary tuberculosis.
(b) Open tuberculosis with caseous pus from a sinus of the internal mammary lymph gland chain. (Typical appearance of caseous pus and indolent lividity of the sinus edges.) A pacemaker has been implanted under the pectoralis major.

81 (a) Hypertrophied gums.
(b) Scurvy — bleeding gums may produce confusion; periodontal disease.
(c) Leukaemia; phenytoin; nifedipine.

82 (a) Acute gout.
(b) Thiazide prescribed for hypertension, blocks excretion of uric acid and leads to hyperuricaemia; advised to lose weight, he becomes ketotic and blocks excretion of uric acid; alcoholic debauch, leads to ketosis, acidosis and precipitation of acute gout.

83 (a) She is acromegalic with a high circulating level of growth hormone increasing the basal metabolic rate, leading to excess sweating in 60 per cent. Note the fleshy nose, prominence of the glabellar ridges and the big lower lip.
(b) Because of median nerve compression in the carpal tunnel secondary to soft tissue overgrowth.
(c) Thyrotoxicosis, acromegaly, hypoglycaemia, phaeochromocytoma, or an anxiety state.

84 (a) Take blood for blood sugar estimation and give intravenous glucose.
(b) Insulin fat atrophy (lipoatrophy); this occurs more commonly than hypertrophy, usually in the first 6 months of treatment. Red plaques and thickened subcutaneous nodules may also occur.
(c) Localised scleroderma and morphoea with loss of subcutaneous tissue, hide-like thickening and pigmentation of the overlying skin. Chronic relapsing panniculitis with painful tender red nodular fat usually on the thigh and buttocks, leaving an atrophic area when it heals.

85–86 (a) Ankylosing spondylitis.
(b) The axial skeleton joint shows inflammation of fibrocartilage with calcification which may affect the spine, sacroiliac joints and the proximal synovial joints. Uveal inflammation leads to uveitis. Aortic inflammation leads to aortic incompetence. HLAB27 is present in 90 per cent of cases associated with inflammatory bowel disease — Crohn's and ulcerative colitis.
(c) Costovertebral and costochondral joint involvement leads to pain and tenderness aggravated by lying down.
(d) Fusion and immobility of the cervical spine with unstable atlantoaxial joints may result in atlantoaxial subluxation and cord compression if stressed by a whiplash injury, as well as difficulty with sideways vision.

87 (a) Olecranon bursitis; nodules on the ulnar border; spindled digits; ulnar deviation of fingers; nicotine staining.
(b) Gouty tophi; rheumatoid arthritis.
(c) Ridging and beading of the nail; splinter haemorrhages; vasculitic changes in the nailfold.
(d) Rheumatoid arthritis.

88 (a) Facial mooning due to sodium and water retention; acne and greasiness of the skin; hirsutes due to adrenal androgens; plethora due to thinning of the skin; polycythaemia and obesity due to increased gluconeogenesis and decreased peripheral glucose utilisation.
(b) Ectopic production of ACTH by a lung tumour; overproduction of ACTH by a pituitary tumour (ACTH-dependent); adrenal carcinoma (ACTH-independent); administration of corticosteroid preparations.
(c) Cushing's syndrome (hyperadrenocorticalism).

89 (a) A right Horner's syndrome — cervical sympathetic lesion with a right-sided ptosis and a small right pupil; gangrene of the fingertips affecting the index and middle on the right and the middle *only* on the left.
(b) Horner's syndrome — right-sided cervical rib, right apical lung tumour, or syringomyelia; gangrene — bilateral Raynaud's phenomenon, bilateral ergotism, or syringomyelia.
(c) The unilateral right Horner's syndrome is on the side with the worst gangrene because a right-sided cervical sympathectomy was performed for severe induced gangrene in a girl who took ergotamine for migraine.

90 (a) Oculogyric crisis.
(b) Spasmodic upward conjugate deviation of the eyes.
(c) Drug-induced phenothiazines; post-encephalitic in Parkinson's disease; epilepsy.

91 (a) The patella may be rudimentary or absent.
(b) The V-shaped lunula, a characteristic feature of the nail patella syndrome of both mesodermal and ectodermal defects.
(c) Defective, small or partially absent ulnar half of the nails; an increased carrying angle at the elbow; iliac horns; albuminuria.
(d) Nail patella syndrome.

92, 93 (a) Acromegaly with an enlarging pituitary tumour interfering with gonadotrophin production and leading to impotence.
(b) Excess growth hormone leads to an increase in sweating and in soft tissue overgrowth. Note the broad spatulate fingers (control on the left), the ridge at the nailfolds due to an increase in flesh — his feet are fleshy, the soles spreading into the interdigital space and requiring larger-size footwear.

94 (a) Keratoconjunctivitis sicca; polyarthritis: lesions of rheumatoid arthritis, systemic lupus erythematosus or scleroderma may all be associated with keratoconjunctivitis and/or xerostomia as Sjögren's syndrome; enlargement due to increased incidence of lymphoma in Sjögren's syndrome; hepatomegaly in association with primary biliary cirrhosis; macrocytosis in association with pernicious anaemia. All these are common associations of the sicca syndrome.
(b) Xerostomia, dry tongue.

95 (a) Systemic sclerosis — note the fat fingers, shiny tight skin and ischaemic fingertips.
(b) Skin — Raynaud's phenomenon may be an early feature in 90 per cent of cases; gut — dysphagia secondary to oesophageal involvement; lung — breathlessness from pulmonary fibrosis and pulmonary hypertension; heart — myocardial fibrosis and cardiac failure; renal — hypertension; musculoskeletal — arthralgia.

96 (a) Fleshy lips due to soft tissue overgrowth; prognathic jaw with overbite, the lower jaw closing in front of the upper.
(b) Cartilage degeneration in osteoarthritis; increased muscle mass with fatigue and cramps; tissue overgrowth and the carpal tunnel syndrome.
(c) Acromegaly.

97 (a) Plaque-like orange lesions of cutaneous xanthelasmata; achilles and extensor tendon xanthomas particularly over the fingers and in the patellar tendons; flexor tendons in the feet may show nodules; foot pulses may be absent.
(b) Arcus cornealis: when present before age 30 it may indicate heterozygous familial hypercholesterolaemia with elevation of low density lipoproteins (LDL) inherited as an autosomal dominant. Overproduction/underclearance in the homozygote; 50 per cent manifest symptoms in early adult life, 75 per cent by middle age.

98, 99 (a) Bilateral drooping of the eyelids, has come on after prolonged upward gazing leads to fatigue. Ptosis is eliminated by edrophonium injection.
(b) Thyrotoxicosis — muscular weakness demands exclusion of myasthenia gravis. A smoker with this weakness may have an oat cell carcinoma of the bronchus. Proximal muscle weakness may come on after exertion, is improved after edrophonium, but unlike true myasthenia the reflexes may be absent or sluggish.
(c) Penicillamine and streptomycin, both of which may induce myasthenia.
(d) Myasthenia gravis.

100 (a) The pupils are equal, there is no external ocular muscle palsy or squint so she either has a right-sided ptosis or a left-sided lid retraction (the contact lenses are irrelevant). With the former she could have a partial IIIrd nerve lesion or a Horner's syndrome, but with weight loss, diarrhoea and sweating the possibility that she was thyrotoxic should be considered by checking the thyroid-stimulating hormone (TSH) response to intravenous TRH.
(b) Right-sided ptosis.

101, 102 (a) Erythema nodosum: nodular vasculitis of the subcutis producing raised bruise-like lumps.
(b) Common causes include: streptococcal infection; primary tuberculosis; pregnancy; contraceptive pill; sulphonamides; leprosy. Less common causes include: cat scratch disease; Epstein–Barr virus infection; mycoplasma; ulcerative colitis; Crohn's disease.
(c) A full history and chest X-ray.

103, 104 (a) A perforating ulcer which may occur in: diabetes or tabes dorsalis, characterised by loss of pain sense; leprosy.
(b) The median and ulnar nerves with trauma and loss of the fingertips, producing a simian hand with thenar and hypothenar wasting.
(c) Tuberculoid leprosy, anaesthetic patches and palpable thickened nerves.

105 (a) Testicular disease; liver disease; carcinoma of the bronchus; thyrotoxicosis; puberty; refeeding after illness; pituitary tumour.
(b) Those interfering with gonadotrophin control: phenothiazines; metoclopramide; isoniazid; cimetidine; tricyclic antidepressants. Antiandrogens: spironolactone. Those increasing the rate of androgen to oestrogen conversion in the periphery: androgens and anabolic steroids.
(c) Gynaecomastia. (Differentiate pseudogynaecomastia due to fat from true increase in mammary tissue.)

106 (a) Calcaneal spurs at the achilles tendon insertion and at the plantar aponeurosis attachment due to a periostitis and subsequent new bone formation.
(b) Rheumatoid arthritis, Reiter's syndrome, ankylosing spondylitis, and psoriatic arthropathy.

107 (a) A right-sided ptosis with a small pupil. The lesion of a partial cervical sympathetic nerve due to involvement by carcinoma of the lung apex.
(b) Small muscle wasting of the hand. This is seen affecting the median side of the hand with wasting of abductor pollicis brevis (median nerve, T1). Hypothenar wasting was also present, thus excluding carpal tunnel compression of the median nerve; the face showed a right-sided ptosis and a small pupil.

108 (a) Onycholysis (separation of the nail from its bed).
(b) Trauma; fungal infection; psoriasis; ischaemia; dermatitis of the digits.

109 (a) The skin shows erythema *ab igne* of the abdomen due to temperature trauma to the skin from a hot water bottle as a chronic counter-irritant. One could deduce that chronic pain is felt in the centre of the abdomen, is worse at night, brought on by lying down, better on sitting or bending due to postural associations with stretching of the posterior parietal peritoneum over the tumour enlargement. A similar erythema *ab igne* is sometimes seen in the small of the back. Weight loss is inevitable.
(b) Erythema *ab igne*. When not on the legs it is an important pointer to underlying organic disease — never accept the diagnosis of irritable bowel syndrome; it is usually carcinoma of pancreas.

110, 111 (a) Subcutaneous neurofibromas.
(b) Giant plexiform neuromas may lead to grotesque deformities, with kyphoscoliosis as a complication.
(c) Peripherally: cutaneous manifestations of five or more café-au-lait hyperpigmented spots, and cutaneous peripheral or spinal nerve root neurofibromas; centrally: epilepsy, mental retardation, cranial nerve tumours, gliomas and meningiomas. Ganglion neuromas, phaeochromocytomas, pathological fractures with pseudoarthroses are features. This autosomal dominant trait seems to be more severe if transmitted by the male.
(d) Neurofibromatosis (von Recklinghausen's disease).

112, 113 Hypothyroidism: the large tongue fills the mouth; the puffy face, hands and feet all regress after 3 months treatment on L-thyroxine.

114, 115 (a) Radial nerve (palsy).
(b) Axilla — the crutch palsy: an inability to extend the elbow (triceps), weak brachioradialis (flexion of the elbow, the muscle being felt at the superior lateral aspect of the antecubital fossa), and weak extensors of the wrist and fingers (wrist drop). The spiral groove of the humerus — due to injection, fracture, pressure over a seat back or operating table, in a deep alcoholic sleep or with an anaesthetic, a

weak brachioradialis in addition to long extensor paralysis. Diabetics may be more prone to the effects of pressure. The forearm — the posterior interosseus may be compressed by a fracture, lipoma or after unfamiliar work (such as driving screws). The extensor radialis escapes, so the hand can be dorsiflex asymmetrically but finger extension is not possible. The only sensory upset is with pressure at the wrist when the cutaneous branch to the first dorsal interspace may be compressed by a watchstrap against the radius, or by a survival suit cuff leading to cheiralgia paraesthetica.

116 (a) Rheumatoid arthritis. This has caused swollen metaphalangeal joints but no ulnar drift; small muscle wasting is a secondary effect of inflammation of adjacent joints.
(b) If the hands are turned over, check if there is thenar median wasting; if not, then the ulnar nerve alone is affected. If thenar, then the cause is either local painful arthritis or a lesion in the T1 root. If unilateral ptosis, look for Horner's syndrome; if bilateral, consider a myopathy dystrophia myotonica. Look for burns of syringomyelia and fasciculation and clawing of the feet in motor neurone disease.
(c) The interossei via the ulnar nerve and T1.

117 (a) Physical trauma by teeth found along the occlusal line of the cheek; pipe smoking; infection — chronic candidiasis and tertiary syphilis; hereditary leuko-keratosis; idiopathic (50 per cent of cases); hairy leukoplakia (Epstein–Barr virus (EBV)-associated) may antedate HIV disease (AIDS).
(b) Leukoplakia (premalignant); white patches are not removed by scraping.
(c) An ulcer with a rolled edge. In 5 per cent of cases this condition is associated with a carcinoma of the tongue which has developed here.

118 (a) It may be a benign congenital oddity.
(b) Heterochromia of the iris.
(c) Posterior lens opacities develop and may need cataract extraction. Hetero-chromia may occur after three or four attacks of uveitis, usually in women, with no underlying cause and unassociated with posterior synechiae. As the pigment falls out, the pupils become green to grey.

119 (a) Tuberculous phlyctenular keratoconjunctivitis, a condition associated with primary infection and tuberculous allergic hypersensitivity. A grey nodule at 8 o'clock with a leash of vessels crossing the limbus is present; nodules may be multiple and recur.
(b) Chest X-ray may show hilar gland enlargement, and the old tuberculin skin test will be positive.
(c) Erythema nodosum and tuberculides — papular necrotic symmetrical granu-lomatous lesions seen on the skin, often of the limbs — are associated with positive tuberculin testing.

120–124 (a) Diabetes mellitus; brain encephalitis; pinealoma; Adie's syndrome. At rest the right pupil is regular, dilated and larger than its fellow — exposure to a bright light produces a brisk reaction on the left and nothing on the right. This is in contradistinction to the small irregular, unreacting pupil occurring in tertiary syphilis.
(b) Adie's syndrome. The sudden noticing of blurred vision reflects the dilated pupil, which reacts sluggishly to light, accommodates briskly, but stays tonically contracted on looking to the distance.
(c) The Argyll Robertson pupil of tertiary syphilis, which may also be fixed to light, reacts on accommodation but is small and irregular and not tonic.
(d) Glaucoma with synechiae; senile myosis; syphilis.

125 (a) Osteomalacia — vitamin D deficiency, characterised by osteoporosis and the appearance of ribbon-like areas of demineralisation, often bilateral and symmetrical (Looser's zones in the pubic rami).

(b) Females may have increased need of vitamin D, and lack of sunlight may lead to lower vitamin D levels as 90 per cent vitamin D is synthesised in the skin (the darkness of her skin is unimportant as controls — negroes — may have normal levels). Custom may cause her to cover herself. A diet high in phytate and fibre may lead to binding of calcium but not vitamin D. The enterohepatic circulation of vitamin D metabolites after its two hydroxylations in the liver and kidney may lead to the active vitamin being trapped in the high fibre content of the gut contents, excluding it from the body and tipping the balance to deficiency. Barbiturates are potent hepatic oxidase inducers which could reduce levels of vitamin D metabolites.

126 (a) Herpes zoster (T2 dermatome).

(b) The character of the pain might have stimulated a search for sensory changes in the T2 area.

(c) On the trunk, more than the limbs, for the trunk has more dermatomes. It usually affects the sensory roots but motor paralysis may occur leading to facial palsy, limb weakness or bladder retention.

127–129 (a) Erythema multiforme, with target-like lesions and a central blister affecting the hands, feet, mouth and genitalia, the Stevens–Johnson syndrome. Ulceration may occur.

(b) For about a month: Beau's lines are noted on the nail, and the nails grow out at the rate of about ½ mm/day.

(c) After herpes simplex; following streptococcal and mycoplasma infections; with sulphonamides; with a neoplasm; in collagen diseases (SLE, rheumatoid arthritis and ulcerative colitis).

130 (a) Sublingual venous engorgement.

(b) Downwards to bypass the superior vena cava; dilated veins may be noted over the upper thorax.

(c) Superior vena caval obstruction.

(d) Enlarged lymph glands as due to neoplasm, usually carcinoma of the bronchus. Rarely aortic aneurysm may compress the vena cava, associated with oedema of the arms, and hoarseness due to left vocal nerve palsy secondary to left recurrent laryngeal nerve compression.

131 (a) Optic atrophy; external ocular palsy; visual field defect; deafness; median nerve palsy.

(b) An increase in soft tissues, tufting of the terminal phalanges, and widening of the joint space.

(c) Wasting of the thenar eminence, particularly the abductor pollicis brevis secondary to the carpal tunnel syndrome.

(d) Acromegaly: broad spatulate fingers and a widening of soft tissues are seen.

(e) A reduction of gonadotrophin secretion by the enlarging tumour.

(f) An increase in metabolic rate.

132 (a) Barium swallow to exclude an oesophageal neoplasm.

(b) Hyperkeratosis of the soles and thickening of the palms associated with: friction; as part of tylosis (familial defect, associated with hyperkeratosis of the palms and carcinoma of the oesophagus); drugs (practolol, as part of a syndrome of dry eyes, skin rash and plastic peritonitis); psoriasis; secondary syphilis; Reiter's disease (keratoderma blenorrhagica).

133 (a) Hyperalgesia over the area of the rash.
(b) C2; C1 has no sensory supply in the head and the rash spares the pretragal area (supplied by the maxillary branch of the Vth nerve).
(c) Herpes zoster.

134 (a) Chickenpox. Crops of macular, papular and vesicular lesions present at all stages. The varicella zoster virus shows a centripetal distribution compared to smallpox or erythema multiforme. In a child the prodrome may be very mild.
(b) Varicella zoster affecting the nerves, a reactivation of a previous varicella infection when the level of varicella zoster neutralising antibody disappears; it usually persists for 40 years thus accounting for its appearance at 50+. Epidemics of chickenpox may occur, but never of herpes zoster.
(c) Secondary infection of the lung with a severe bronchopneumonia or a mild pneumonia, but residual miliary calcification seen on chest X-ray. Hepatitis, as a hepatocellular jaundice. Encephalitis, with headache. Purpura fulminans.

135 (a) Rheumatoid arthritis in the hand (classic deformity).
(b) Gamekeeper's thumb — caused by volar subluxation of the first metacarpophalangeal joint with rupture of the medial collateral ligament.
(c) Swan-neck or grasshopper deformity of the finger occurs due to contraction of the lumbrical and interossei muscles leading to hyperextension of the proximal interphalangeal joints, the muscles working as extensors rather than flexors. Erosion of the extensor tendon may lead to a permanently flexed distal interphalangeal joint.

136, 137 (a) Hypothyroidism produces a characteristic change in the hair of the hands and shins, rather like mown stubble, which regrows after treatment. Similar appearances may occur with chronic debilitating diseases, ischaemia of a limb, or chemotherapy, although in the latter two total loss of hair is more common.
(b) Alopecia of myxoedema.

138 (a) Terminal interphalangeal joint swelling may be bony, caused by degenerative joint disease and Heberden's nodes, or by joint swelling in psoriatic arthritis (5 per cent). Pitting of the fingernails on the lateral border of the index is seen.
(b) Psoriatic arthritis.

139 (a) Herpes genitalis, after rupture of the vesicle, a sexually transmitted disease caused by type II herpes virus in 90 per cent; recurrences are often associated with pain in the sacral segments.
(b) Gonorrhoea, syphilis and lymphogranuloma venereum should be excluded.
(c) Introspection and anxiety; in the pregnant female may lead to herpes (type II virus) infection of the neonate; infestation of a cervix with herpes may be a factor in carcinoma of the cervix.

140 (a) Chickenpox may be distinguished from smallpox by the fact that the former affects the axilla. The freckles of von Recklinghausen's disease may be seen initially in the axilla in a child prior to being manifest elsewhere, but are uncommon in the shaded area of the axilla. Eczema and dermatitis may be more common in the axilla, as may scabies at its edge. Acanthosis nigricans should be distinguished from pseudo-acanthosis nigricans, more common in obese people.
(b) Varicella zoster is noted in the apex of the axilla with vesicles on an erythematous base. Careful examination shows a further rash spreading round in the T2 dermatome over the pectoralis muscle and the nipple.

141 (a) Lid retraction, a white rim of sclera seen around the eye, combined with shininess of the skin due to sweating because of increased heat production related to the rise in metabolic rate.

(b) Lidlag, proptosis and external ocular palsy.

(c) Thyrotoxicosis.

(d) Myasthenia gravis may occur more often than expected. Proximal muscle weakness may be a presenting complaint with difficulty on going up stairs or driving a bus. Increasing fatigue with exercise and relief with rest may be seen with diplopia or ptosis.

142 (a) Raynaud's disease. Ischaemic changes are seen in the index finger due to primary digital arterial vasospasm leading to pallor, cyanosis and erythema, occasionally progressing to gangrene of the tip.

(b) Drugs (ergotamine, methysergide); arterial obstruction — cervical rib, pressure from an axillary crutch producing embolic phenomena; trauma — vibrating tools associated with connective tissue diseases; cryoglobulins producing cold agglutinins.

143 Hypothyroidism with macroglossia and the carpal tunnel syndrome; acromegaly with an enlarged fleshy tongue and the carpal tunnel syndrome; amyloid infiltration of the tongue and nerves. Macroglossia may also be seen in Down's syndrome and as a congenital lone abnormality.

144 (a) Galactorrhoea.

(b) Prolactin. A high level is associated with impotence.

(c) Stress (of venepuncture); sleep; nipple stimulation; coitus; pregnancy; suckling.

(d) Increased secretion may be produced by a pituitary prolactinoma. A non-secreting pituitary tumour may physically interfere with the hypothalamic dopamine-mediated inhibition of normal production. Drugs blocking dopamine receptors (metoclopramide and phenothiazines) lead to increased production. Drugs depleting brain dopamine (alphamethyldopa and reserpine) produce less marked elevation. Hypothyroidism. Ectopic production by non-endocrine tumours. Note: in liver disease there is an increase in oestrogens which leads to gynaecomastia only, as does spironolactone.

145 (a) An acute monoarthritis of gout involving the midtarsus (a common site, although less typical than the great toe) caused pain preventing sleep.

(b) To exclude a stress fracture.

(c) Although no trauma had occurred, unaccustomed exertion may explain the localisation of the arthritis to the foot. Alcohol excess may lead to ketosis, preventing excretion of uric acid, and hyperuricaemia which may precipitate the attack.

146 (a) Ankylosing spondylitis.

(b) HLAB27 histocompatibility: 90 per cent of patients with ankylosing spondylitis are HLAB27 positive with a higher incidence in their families. Crohn's colitis and sacroiliitis may also be associated with HLAB27.

(c) Fusion of vertebrae along the anterior spinal ligament giving rise to 'bamboo' spine.

(d) Uveitis (also associated with HLAB27); aortitis (may lead to aortic incompetence); apical lung fibrosis with cavitation.

147 (a) A right ptosis with a small pupil and a sunken eye.

(b) Horner's syndrome — paralysis of the cervical sympathetic, full syndrome consisting of enophthalmos (rarely obvious), and loss of sweating on the affected side with a small pupil and right ptosis.

(c) Apical lung tumour involving the brachial plexus giving pain in the hand.

148 (a) Localised scleroderma with atrophy of the upper limb, particularly affecting the skin and subcutaneous muscles and tissues leading to contracture of the hand. It may be associated with hemiatrophy and plaques of morphoea, one of which can be seen on the right hand on the ulnar border of the wrist.
(b) It does not lead to systemic involvement and general health remains good.

149 (a) Serum lipid estimations. Nodules are seen in the achilles tendon of the left heel and with a family history of a young myocardial infarction, may indicate tendon xanthomata in familial hypercholesterolaemia.
(b) Extensor tendons of the hands and the skin of the eyelids may also show lipid deposit; a similar appearance is also seen at the heel in runners due to shoe friction, and in rheumatoid arthritis, rheumatic fever and rarely as gouty tophi.

150 (a) Coup de sabre — local scleroderma of linear distribution, with atrophy of subcutaneous tissues which may affect the face with sclerosis of subcutaneous tissues and associated hemiatrophy.
(b) Yes. There are no systemic manifestations and it does not progress.
(c) Skin thickening, which is hard, hide-like and pigmented — local morphoea — and occurs in plaques. By contrast, progressive scleroderma is a systemic disease (multiple system involvement) associated with tightening of the skin in Raynaud's phenomenon; it may affect the gut, lung, kidney and joints.

151, 152 (a) Pigmented gums.
(b) Racial in dark-skinned persons; secondary to tattooing — cosmetic tattooing occurs in Sudan and Ethiopia, and therapeutic tattooing disguised as cosmetic tattoo to strengthen the left first upper incisor injured in a fall. Note the dark incisor and alternative pattern added so that unsightly tattoo marks are disguised. Addison's disease with excess ACTH from the pituitary leads to pigmentation over pressure areas, of exposed parts of the body, scars, and particularly of the gums and buccal mucosa; also in Nelson's syndrome, due to very high ACTH levels from a pituitary tumour, where there is no feedback response from high cortisol levels.

153 (a) The legs are oedematous, with palpable red inflamed veins seen particularly on the inside of the right knee caused by venous thrombosis.
(b) Thrombophlebitis migrans.
(c) Malignancy, which may declare itself later usually with carcinoma of the pancreas.

154 (a) Alopecia areata.
(b) Patchy alopecia, due to secondary syphilis; scarring alopecia, due to discoid lupus; ringworm (no scales); trauma and hair pulling leading to bald patches.
(c) Atopy, sickle cell disease and Down's syndrome all have an increased frequency of alopecia areata. There is poor prognosis in the first two.
(d) Nails may be ridged and pitted; vitiligo.
(e) Exclamation mark hairs (seen as black dots): damage weakens the hair in the keratogenous zone and precipitates it into catagen — the hair breaks when the keratogenous zone reaches the surface.

155 (a) The medical outpatients' diabetic clinic.
(b) Hypoglycaemia (produced by excess insulin), shown by aggression combined with profuse sweating, coldness of extremities and tachycardia.
(c) Alcohol taken on an empty stomach may inhibit gluconeogenesis in the fasting state; liver glycogen stores are depleted inducing hypoglycaemia.

156 (a) Haemochromatosis.
(b) The skin is pigmented — a grey colour due to excess melanin compared to the control hand on the left — and may coexist with a severe degenerative arthropathy. In ochronosis (alcaptonuria) the colour change is confined to cartilage and is then seen as a grey discoloration through the skin. In both conditions X-ray may show a degenerative arthropathy with chondrocalcinosis at a young age.
(c) Chondrocalcinosis and degenerative joint disease affecting the metacarpo-interphalangeal joint, hips and knees.
(d) Osteoarthritis, hyperparathyroidism, gout, pseudogout and Wilson's disease.

157–160 (a) Flat expressionless face of Parkinson's disease: staring eyes, sweaty from tremor and rigidity due to dopamine-depleted substantia nigra **(157)**. Jaundice, cholestatic hepatitis B, often associated with itch producing polishing of the fingernails **(158)**. Violaceous plaque on the skin in a young air steward (Kaposi's sarcoma) **(159)**. Haemosiderin tattooed into the skin in a mainlining heroin drug addict **(160)**.
(b) The tattoo of a drug addict **(160)** who can develop: hepatitis B **(158)**, or AIDS (Kaposi's sarcoma of the skin in HIV infection) **(159)**, or Parkinson's syndrome **(157)** if his heroin is contaminated by methyl phenyl tetra pyridine (MPTP) which wipes out the substantia nigra dopamine.

161 (a) Anaphylactoid non-thrombocytopaenic purpura, seen here as cutaneous vasculitis (Henoch–Schönlein purpura) secondary to immune complex formation with IgA deposition, and may involve renal, cutaneous and intestinal vessels.
(b) Polyarthralgia with a migrating transient large joint discomfort; haematuria and proteinuria secondary to a proliferative glomerulonephritis in 50 per cent of cases with IgA seen in the glomerular capillaries; gut involvement secondary to inflammation with colic, bleeding and intersussception; a skin rash (the spectrum runs from urticarial wheals to a purpuric rash affecting the limbs and buttocks associated with vesiculation).
(c) Upper respiratory tract infections (30 per cent streptococcal); drugs (penicillin, sulphonamides, benzothiadiazides); vascular purpuras in rickettsial and meningo-coccal infections.

162 (a) Myxoedema. Hypothyroidism with coarse apathetic facies and thickened soft tissue features, all reverting to normal with L-thyroxine replacement.
(b) Alopecia (like stubble on a cornfield); limb oedema, giving a characteristic puffiness; cool and dry skin; the palms have yellow-to-white colour secondary to a normochromic anaemia and betacarotenaemia in hypothyroidism.
(c) Carpal tunnel compression of the median nerve (a common complication of myxoedema); symmetrical sensory neuropathy of all four limbs, responding to L-thyroxine; occasionally associated extensor plantars may suggest a demyelinating cord component and about 12.5 per cent myxoedema patients may also have pernicious anaemia, paraesthesiae being a manifestation of vitamin B_{12} deficiency.

163, 164 (a) Liver palms and soles.
(b) Morning nausea associated with gastritis of alcoholism; cirrhosis of the liver; vitamin B deficiency; pregnancy.
(c) White nails (also seen in cirrhosis, chronic congestive cardiac failure, and non-insulin dependent diabetes mellitus); Dupuytren's contracture (may be seen in alcoholics, with nodules in the plantar fascia); spider naevi — a feeding arteriole into radiating capillaries is associated with liver disease, but may also be seen in pregnancy, appearing in the first month and subsiding in the first week postpartum; distribution is usually in superior vena cava drainage. Hair loss.

165 (a) Thyrotoxicosis.

(b) Lid retraction — the right eye also shows some proptosis, not obvious from this view; sweating — skin is warm, moist and glistening; tension and irritability — patient's complaint of a short temper shows in the tense facies.

(c) Lidlag; ophthalmoplegia and double vision; proptosis; corneal ulceration and keratitis; optic nerve compression.

(d) Auricular fibrillation and cardiac failure in the elderly (cardiovascular changes may overshadow the increase in basal metabolic rate); proximal myopathy and weakness in pedestrians, and golfers and bus drivers (using shoulders); apathy, lethargy and weight loss mimicking depression; diarrhoea and weight loss mimicking an anxiety state.

166 (a) Enlargement of the costochondral junction due to uncalcified osteoid in vitamin D deficiency — 'the rickety rosary'.

(b) Gluten enteropathy (coeliac disease) and steatorrhoea, leading to a loss of vitamin D and calcium in the stool.

(c) Rickets may be nutritional, due to malabsorption or renal disease. The sick mucosa is unable to absorb calcium even in response to the changes produced in RNA by endogenously produced 125-dihydroxycholecalciferol (DHCC).

167, 168 (a) Herpes zoster, due to activation in the dorsal root ganglion of latent varicella zoster virus leading to pain in nerve distribution.

(b) Dysaesthesiae over the dermatome affected, prior to the rash appearance. The characteristic vesicular rash seen in the loin may spread over the dermatome, limited to the midline.

(c) A surgical gridiron incision may be superimposed on the rash if appendicitis cannot be excluded!

169–171 (a) 'Wet' cupping — practised throughout Europe and the Middle East — the application of warm glass vessels which adhere to the skin (wet, as the skin is excoriated first to allow 'bad toxic blood' egress, and often used in respiratory disease). 'Dry' cupping is without scarification.

(b) A shearing rupture of the epigastric artery in the rectus abdominus produces a mass (easily seen on ultrasound examination, **171**) in the upper abdomen if the superior epigastric artery, and the lower abdomen with the inferior epigastric artery, with pain worse on contraction of the abdominal muscles when the lump may disappear as it lies behind the muscle and mimics an intra-abdominal mass.

(c) Shearing stress (ruptured inferior epigastric artery, fractured rib — the upper thorax moves in and the lower thorax moves out and a fatigue fracture can occur at the site of shearing); obstruction to venous return (cardiac output falls and syncope occurs); capillary rupture with purpura; subconjunctival haemorrhage; an increase in abdominal pressure leading to hernia, incontinence, vomiting; cough headache — a rise in intracranial pressure leading to sudden pain lasting for 10 minutes and subsiding, rarely complicated by intracranial bleeding.

172–174 (a) Kaposi's sarcoma.

(b) African variety is an aggressive invasive tumour characterised by violaceous skin plaques, black under negro skin, ultimately fatal (**172**). Classic Kaposi's sarcoma, first described in Jews, is indolent, confined to the skin, may be present for decades, death being caused by unrelated disease (**173**). AIDS-associated variety has plum-coloured violet plaques on the skin, mouth and palate, appearing in crops on the limbs; rapidly fatal, more common in sexually acquired AIDS (**174**).

(c) Acquired immune deficiency syndrome due to HIV infection, affecting either sex, more common in certain high-risk groups where blood contamination is possible — transfusions in haemophiliacs, syringes in drug addicts, from anal and vaginal intercourse — the common factor being multiple sexual partners rather than hetero/homosexuality.

175 (a) Perniosis or chilblains of the toes, a cold-induced ischaemia secondary to a combination of tight shoes occluding the blood supply and poor insulation, common in winter in temperate climates. Chilblains are a cutaneous vasculitis with liberation of histamine, itch, inflammation and ischaemia.
(b) Tight jeans with the insulation produced by fat thighs may lead to ischaemic cold skin injury of the thighs, the skin becoming pink, blue and mottled (cutis marmorata); acrocyanosis with a pink/blue hand; venostasis in cold extremities may account for the peripheral distribution of many rashes as immune complexes may be trapped, causing damage; Raynaud's phenomenon may be induced by cold.

176 (a) Sickle cell disease.
(b) Osteomyelitis with a huge sequestrum — so-called bone within a bone.
(c) *Salmonella typhi.*

177 (a) Rheumatoid arthritis; ischaemic sores over pressure areas of the foot in an individual with rheumatoid arthritis, cutaneous vasculitis and rheumatic nodules occur in areas of pressure and cooling which predisposes to venostasis, immune complex trapping and consequent vessel injury.
(b) By well-fitting shoes and adequate insulation.

178 The man is a Muslim. There is an area of hyperkeratinisation in the central forehead, caused by friction of the forehead against the ground while praying. Problems of drug compliance and insulin dose in diabetics may arise during the fasting month of Ramadan.

179 (a) Hypothyroidism.
(b) Menorrhagia, which may precipitate anaemia (secondary amenorrhoea may also occur in hypothyroidism); blood loss secondary to bleeding haemorrhoids caused by straining at stool; thyroxine deficiency, which may lead to a normochromic normocytic anaemia correcting with replacement therapy; macrocytic anaemia due to concomitant vitamin B_{12} deficiency of pernicious anaemia more frequently associated with hypothyroidism. Her haemoglobin corrected on replacement therapy with L-thyroxine and oral iron.

180 (a) Neuropathic joint (painless abnormal range of movement of the knee).
(b) Syringomyelia, picking off the crossing fibres of the spinothalamic tracts and rendering the hands anaesthetic; leprosy, leading to a peripheral neuropathy and loss of sensation.
(c) Diabetes mellitus in the ankle joint; tabes dorsalis; spina bifida.

181 (a) Neuropathic ankle joint.
(b) Warmth due to increased blood flow; diminished sensation due to neuropathy; abnormal range of movement leading to joint destruction; absent ankle jerk due to a break in the reflex arc.
(c) Due to an autonomic neuropathy there is increased shunting of blood, seen as an increased flow in the veins: the foot will be warm and there is osteoporis due to the increased blood flow; minor trauma may lead to bony collapse with subsequent inflammation and joint destruction further aggravated by poor sensation.
(d) Joint destruction due to osteoporosis.

(e) Syringomyelia, usually upper limb neuropathic joint unassociated with pain; tabes dorsalis; leprosy.

182 In the lower finger severe growth arrest occurred just after the large splinter haemorrhage with erythema multiforme. A ridge/depression is present halfway up the nail which appears with impaired nail growth during an acute illness or local limb ischaemia. The time elapsed since the event can be estimated as 8 weeks earlier as fingernails grow at the rate of about ½ mm/week.

183 (a) Tetanus.
(b) In this emotionally bland face the striking feature is the contracted sternomastoid muscles seen in conditions where there is increase in muscle rigidity, particularly Parkinson's disease and tetanus (where there may be no history of preceding injury). Tonic contraction of the sternomastoids is due to increasing stiffness in the muscles, agonist and antagonist groups, leading to difficulty in opening the mouth and paucity of movement, interspersed with spasms.
(c) Respiratory failure due to increasing rigidity, and intermittent laryngeal spasm associated with cardiovascular instability due to autonomic involvement. During the early phases (first 2–3 days), anxiety, tachycardia, stiffness and twitching may be misinterpreted as functional disease.

184 (a) Lichen planus which may be intensely itchy, appear as a rash at the ankles, around the wrist, over the penis and inside the mouth, and cause depigmentation (as here).
(b) Trauma associated with scarring. Vitiligo, a major trauma in a dark-skinned community because of the problems of the lesion, and frequent complaint in dermatological clinics in Africa. Lichen sclerosis atrophicans which may affect the perineum, causing thinning of the skin and depigmentation. Venous eczema due to varicose veins; no varicose veins are noted and the flat raised plaques of lichen planus are seen.
(c) Tuberculoid leprosy (remember to test sensation over the lesion).

185 (a) Omit alcohol, aspirin or prostaglandin synthetase inhibitors given for degenerative joint disease.
(b) Campbell de Morgan spots (cherry red vascular malformations); in the ageing skin with scleroderma; radiotherapy; in Fabry disease, when there may be angiokeratomata seen particularly over the buttocks.
(c) Osler–Weber–Rendu disease (hereditary telangiectasia), usually presenting late in life with anaemia and nose bleeds (after 40 years of age).

186 (a) Lidlag is seen — spastic lid retraction is a common eye sign in thyrotoxicosis, present in all gaze positions and confirmed when the cornea becomes visible as the eye follows an examining finger downwards from a position of upward gaze. In myotonia congenita and dystrophia myotonica, if the gaze is fixed for a few moments and then the eyes depressed suddenly, there is a dramatic lidlag.
(b) Lidlag in myotonia — failure to relax levator palpebri superioris as the eyes are moved downwards; hand grip may be slow to relax especially in the cold, which aggravates the myotonia. Percussion over a muscle may elicit a dimple of contraction which persists for several seconds. In dystrophia myotonica this may be seen long before muscle wasting is obvious.

187 (a) Tuberculous lymphadenitis, the primary focus being in the tonsils and the neck showing multiple sinuses with characteristic violaceous change in the skin. Abscesses are both superficial and deep to the fascia (collarstud).

(b) A hypersensitivity reaction of phlyctenular keratoconjunctivitis.

(c) Bovine mycobacterium, less common in the United Kingdom because of tuberculin testing and pasteurisation; in developing countries, where there is no milk, bovine tuberculosis is less common but it occurs in areas where milk is available and hygiene is poor.

(d) Small intestine and mesenteric lymph nodes may lead to primary abdominal tuberculosis and tuberculous peritonitis or perianal sinuses.

188 (a) Psoriatic oligoarticular arthritis (the most common form of arthropathy in psoriasis — 70 per cent of cases) and tenosynovitis. This form is less striking than the symmetrical distal interphalangeal joint enlargement being asymmetrical, usually affecting the metacarpophalangeal and proximal interphalangeal joints, flexor tenosynovitis producing a sausage digit appearance.

(b) Short-term swelling — gout, trauma, sickle cell disease, bone infarct; long-term swelling — sausage digit of psoriasis, gouty tophi, sarcoid bone cysts (look for lupus pernio), Ollier's disease (enchondroplasia), and chronic inflammation such as tuberculosis and syphilitic gummata.

189 (a) Partial unilateral ptosis with a downward, outward-looking eye due to the unopposed action of the superior oblique and lateral rectus. The pupil is not seen. There is therefore a IIIrd nerve palsy, which may occur in migraine and be recurrent and transient.

(b) A IIIrd nerve palsy may be: nuclear — disseminated sclerosis, mid-brain neoplasm, syphilis; mid-brain — vascular, posterior cerebral artery thrombosis; interpeduncular — aneurysm, syphilis, tuberculosis, fracture, posterior communicating artery aneurysm, raised intracranial pressure; cavernous sinus — aneurysm or fistula; the orbit — tumour or fracture; rarely in association with diabetes mellitus.

190 (a) XIIth (wasting of the left side of the tongue).

(b) At the base of the skull (shown by left-sided ptosis due to a sympathetic lesion).

(c) Tumours at the base of the skull may be benign neurofibromata, or reflect the high incidence of nasopharyngeal carcinoma in southern China.

191 (a) Left. The left ankle has a disorganised mortice joint; the right is normal.

(b) A neuropathic joint in insulin-dependent diabetes mellitus, which should occur on the non-hemiplegic side, subject to greater trauma.

192 (a) Pitted nails grow faster than normal nails, growth being between 0.5 and 1.2 mm/week. The longer fingers have the fastest nail growth and the right hand tends to grow faster than the left. Growth may slow down with illness in association with the yellow nail syndrome, growth arrest may occur, or Beau's lines may be present. Toenails grow at about half the rate of fingernails.

(b) In normal people; in alopecia areata; with psoriasis; with fungus infections; with chronic paronychia.

193 (a) Whether he is homosexual; HIV antibody test.

(b) Hairy leukoplakia — papilliferous leukoplakia associated with Epstein-Barr virus genome incorporation, common AIDS and in association with squamous carcinoma; Kaposi tumour in the mouth and palate.

(c) Lichen planus and leukoplakia but in oral candidiasis wiping discloses a red base. Oral and oesophageal candida may be associated with: infancy; old age, particularly at the angles of the mouth where absorption of the teeth leads to overclosure of the bite and a soggy area; dentures; antibiotic therapy with a change in bacterial flora; cytotoxic drugs; diseases with impaired immune response — leukaemia and infection with HIV; AIDS, and ARC, in both of which it may be the first sign or presenting feature.

194 (a) Protein energy malnutrition.
(b) Small intestinal bacterial overgrowth leads to fermentation and malabsorption.
(c) Oedema, secondary to sodium/water (Na/H_2O) retention; hyperpigmentation with a cracking and peeling skin, lacking inflammatory response, possibly related to zinc deficiency; depigmentation and loss of the hair; hepatic enlargement.
(d) Midstream urine to screen for urinary infection; blood films for malarial parasites; stools for ova; cysts and parasites; fundoscopy for retinal tubercules and a chest X-ray for tuberculosis.

195 (a) Alcohol (which may induce flushing, as may heat, emotion or exercise); sugar: type II non-insulin-dependent diabetes mellitus individuals may inherit a tendency to flush with alcohol when taking chlorpropamide. The inheritance is Mendelian dominant, and there is a lower incidence of retinopathy; 5-hydroxyindole acetic acid: flushing is the classic symptom of the carcinoid syndrome affecting the head and neck and associated with a tachycardia, diarrhoea or wheezing.
(b) Ultraviolet light exposure; menopause; open air; cholinergic urticaria; steroids; rosacea; lupus pernio; dermatomyositis; disseminated lupus erythematosus.

196 (a) Risus sardonicus, a fixed sardonic smile or grin due to rigid spasm of the facial muscles at the angle of the mouth, with flared alae nasi, and eyelids raised but with absence of mirth. The contracted sustained rigidity in a case of severe tetanus of a spasm precipitated by a slamming door.
(b) Tetanus, as part of a generalised background rigidity on which spasms are superimposed; strychnine poisoning; phenothiazine overdosage and facial dyskinesia (but then associated with trismus and episodes of mouth opening); hysteria; catalepsy; tetany.

197 (a) Staining caused by holding a wad of chewing tobacco in the buccal sulcus.
(b) Neoplasia (early leukoplakia has occurred).

198, 199 (a) Psoriatic arthritis with sacroiliitis. The nails show onycholysis and pitting, associated with an increased frequency of HLAB27.
(b) The skin of the penis may be one of the hidden areas for psoriasis when the individual denies a rash; the scalp, perineum, natal cleft and umbilicus.
(c) Onycholysis may be found in psoriasis, fungus infection, drugs, ischaemia, thyroid disease and dermatitis, and there is also an idiopathic variety.

200 (a) Salivary gland tumour; enlarged lymph glands — reticulosis; tuberculosis (as in this case); branchial cyst, in which the lump will peep out from the upper third of the sternomastoid.
(b) Lymphoma.

201 There is increased pigmentation, particularly around the knuckles which does not extend to areas covered by her rings. She suffers from Addison's disease and developed pigmentation in the preceding year. This is related to an increased secretion of ACTH. Another patient may present with a similar picture following treatment for ACTH-dependent hyperadrenocorticalism, secondary to pituitary tumour and adrenal hyperplasia. After treatment by adrenalectomy alone, ACTH levels will remain elevated and pigmentation will occur (Nelson's syndrome).

202, 203 (a) I^{131} for hyperthyroidism — a treated thyrotoxic — 50 per cent may develop hypothyroidism.
(b) Because of the development of pretibial myxoedema (PTM) over the shin and dorsum of the foot.
(c) This may occur from thyrotoxic ocular myopathy, frequently associated with pretibial myxoedema, and a high incidence of long-acting thyroid stimulator antibody. It typically occurs after treatment with I^{131} and may accompany early hypothyroidism.

204, 205 (a) Lower motor neurone VIIth nerve palsy; myasthenia gravis.
(b) In the first, the orbicularis oris to make a seal and prevent dribbling. (Note the left lower and upper facial weakness — the left eye rolls up and the right face moves. This palsy usually indicates a lesion between the nucleus and the canal portion of the nerve.) In the second, there is bilateral weakness. The mouth hangs open because a weak jaw needs to be supported. There is an inability to shut both eyes and both the facial and jaw muscles are weak and tired. When asked to show the teeth a myasthenic snarl appears due to orbicularis oris weakness.

206 (a) Dilated veins related to an autonomic neuropathy with increased flow, vascular shunting, which may lead to osteoporosis. Oedema may be found in the foot (which will be warm and dry from impaired sweating) as a consequence of the flow.
(b) By an increase in friction, callouses, perforating ulcers, osteoporosis, neuropathic joints, all of which may be aggravated by the poor sensation and blood supply.
(c) Diabetic autonomic neuropathy.
(d) Gastroparesis; postural hypotension; loss of cardiac denervation and a high resting heart rate; impotence; sweating abnormalities.

207 (a) Necrobiosis lipoidica.
(b) Sugar, for this disease was first described in association with diabetes mellitus (3/1000 diabetics may have this condition). It also occurs in the normal population, and may precede diabetes mellitus by some years. There is usually an indurated plaque with central atrophy similar to granuloma annulare.
(c) Fungal and bacterial infections, Dupuytren's contracture, acanthosis nigricans, and lichen planus are all more common in the diabetic and their presence is a prompt to test the urine.

208 (a) Specific anaerobic cultures were not performed.
(b) Metronidazole, which may prevent the dramatic tissue necrosis occurring with anaerobic infection.
(c) Anaerobic infection has a characteristic smell.

209 (a) Cold: the anatomy of the skin leads to thickening and mottling known as cutis marmorata; if chronic the appearance may be that of livido reticularis. Heat: a similar appearance may be produced, also related to the skin circulation and occurring on the surface exposed to fire or hot water bottle; known as erythema *ab igne*.

(b) Livido reticularis on limbs may occur in peripheral vascular disease, or may indicate an underlying neoplasm.

210 (a) Dermatomyositis.
(b) A rash over the dorsum and the knuckles, scaly atrophic lesions (collodion patches which are dark on a pigmented skin and violet in a pale skin). There is pigmentation also in the nailfolds with a vasculitis, and there is a similar appearance on the dorsum of the feet and knees.
(c) A periorbital heliotrope discoloration and oedema.

211 (a) Guinea worm *(Dracunculus medinensis)*. It has failed to gain access to water and therefore has died. It would be eradicated if one had uncontaminated water for all, because the free-swimming cerciae would no longer have access to the body.
(b) Curled-up calcified worms.

212 (a) A DNA papovavirus.
(b) They are capillaries at the tips of elongated papillae.
(c) Lymphoma; immunosuppression; infection with human immunodeficiency virus (HIV), causing acquired immune deficiency syndrome (AIDS).

213 (a) Any childhood illness, particularly malaria.
(b) The swelling pushing the left ear forwards — the appearance of an acute mastoiditis secondary to otitis media.
(c) Cerebellar brain abscess.
(d) Left mastoiditis.

214 (a) The extensor aspect of the finger joints, achilles tendon and the occiput, as they are all characterised by chronic inflammation in subcutaneous tissue usually secondary to mechanical pressure. In rheumatoid arthritis 20 per cent of patients may show chronic inflammatory nodules over bony prominences.
(b) Nodules combined with ulnar drift of the fingers.
(c) Rheumatoid nodules in rheumatoid arthritis, rheumatic fever, gouty tophi, xanthomata in lipid disorders, amyloidosis.

215 (a) Upper cervical lymphadenopathy; salivary gland tumour, although one would expect this to be more anterior; branchial cyst which would transilluminate and peep out from behind the upper third of the sternomastoid; laryngocele, which would increase in size with expiration against a closed glottis.
(b) Branchial cyst as it appears from behind the upper third of the sternomastoid, and transillumines.

216 (a) The free edges of both fingernails are broken suggesting brittle nails; they are dystrophic, and have some concavity; all these suggest iron deficiency.
(b) The vasculitic lesion present in the nailfold is unrelated to iron deficiency and suggests a small vessel inflammation as seen in collagen and immune complex disease.
(c) Disseminated lupus, complicated by the Stevens–Johnson syndrome.

217 (a) Electric shock damage.
(b) A severe electric shock passing through the cord can lead to weakness and progressive wasting, very similar to motor neurone disease. Small muscle wasting of the hand is also seen, either peripheral ulnar neuropathy or a T1 lesion.
(c) Weakness of the feet, clawing of the toes, wasting and exaggerated reflexes, extensor plantars, and fasciculation and wasting of the tongue may show disease of the ventral horn in motor neurone disease affecting both lower and upper motor neurones.

Index